BARRON'S

KEYS TO
DEALING
WITH
CHILDHOOD
ALLERGIES

Judy Lee Bachman, Ph.D.

BARRON'S

All inquiries should be addressed to:
Barron's Educational Series, Inc.
250 Wireless Boulevard
Hauppauge, New York 11788

Library of Congress Catalog Card No. 91-29420

International Standard Book No. 0-8120-4836-9

Library of Congress Cataloging-in-Publication Data

Bachman, Judy Lee.
  Keys to dealing with childhood allergies / Judy Lee Bachman.
     p   cm.—(Barron's parenting keys)
  Includes index.
  ISBN 0-8120-4836-9
  1. Allergy in children—Popular works.   I. Title.   II. Series.
RJ386.B23   1991
618.92'97—dc20   91-29420
                                                                   CIP

PRINTED IN THE UNITED STATES OF AMERICA
2345   5500   987654321

CONTENTS

PREFACE

Allergy is a condition that afflicts 55 million Americans. If both parents have allergies, their children run a strong chance of having allergies as well. It is not unusual for more than one member of a family to have allergies. Allergic diseases are responsible for many days of restricted activity and absences from school or work.

When a child has constant allergy symptoms, he or she may not do as well in play or school. Normal family relations can become difficult. Siblings who do not have allergies may not get the nurturing they need because of the attention that the allergic child requires. The developmental stages of a child can slow down or regress with chronic allergy symptoms.

A marriage can become strained because one or both parents have put too much focus on the allergic child. Sometimes this focus becomes so exaggerated that the child eventually carries the responsibility of holding the family together.

This book introduces allergy and highlights how the parents and their child can become members of the medical team. It provides guidelines to help assure the quality of life of the family.

It is well-known among physicians treating allergy patients that the effectiveness of medical care depends to a great extent upon education of the parents. Education gives parents confidence so they know what to do. With proper education, the desired goals of reduced hospital stays and less time lost from school can be achieved.

Education includes helping the child to take responsibility for his or her health. The parents need to learn how to recognize warning symptoms and triggers. As their children grow, they can teach them how to recognize symptoms. With parental guidance, children will eventually learn when to take action. The youngster will be able to recognize allergens and worsening symptoms.

There have been changes in the treatment of asthma, and it no longer focuses only on spasm of the airways. The basis for asthma is inflammation with phases. To monitor these phases, parents and children use a pulmonary function meter that enables them to make decisions about medications that may avert serious asthma. The treatment medications routine differs in each phase. The environment has also become even more important for children with hypersensitive airways.

It is the intent of this book to introduce an awareness of allergy to parents, teachers, and caregivers so that they will be more understanding of the needs of the allergic child.

1

WHAT IS ALLERGY?

Allergy is an abnormal bodily reaction to substances in the environment. When an allergic person comes in contact with a normally harmless substance, antibodies attach to it, initiating a chain of chemical reactions.

Everyone in the vicinity soon knows when an allergic person comes in contact with certain substances in the environment. The victim will start to sneeze repeatedly or have a runny nose or watery eyes. It was only twenty years ago that researchers found the biological cause of allergies. With the discovery of the antibody IgE, the puzzle began to unravel.

IgE plays an important part in allergy. Some allergy sufferers have a higher level of IgE than other people without allergies. Higher IgE levels tend to run in families; thus it is not unusual to find more than one member of a family with allergies.

The IgE antibody plays a special role. The linings of the respiratory and intestinal tracts have cells to protect the body against foreign particles that may enter it. These cells are called mast cells. One of the places that IgE antibodies reside is on the surface of the mast cells. When a foreign substance (also called antigen or allergen) comes along, the allergen attaches to a specific IgE antibody. The term *specific antibody* means that only one particular substance will attach to it. For example, cat dander is specific to one type of IgE antibody. (See the Glossary for further definition of terms.)

Once the IgE antibody and the allergen attach, a chain of chemical reactions occur. One of the chemicals produced is histamine. With the release of histamine in the nose, for example, the person sneezes and his or her nose runs. Chemicals released from mast cells in the lining of the lower respiratory tract cause asthma. There are many other chemicals involved in the allergy reaction. Research is focused currently on identifying chemicals involved in different phases of asthma.

What is unique about allergies is that no two people have the same allergies or symptoms. One person may get hay fever symptoms from grass, and another may develop asthma. The allergies may change with age from a food allergy to an allergic reaction to pollens, or from hay fever to asthma. They may disappear at puberty and recur during mid-life.

It is not unusual for a child to have gastrointestinal symptoms during the first year or two. Gradually, these symptoms from a food allergy may turn to symptoms from pollen and cause hay fever or asthma around ages 2 to 4. Sometimes the symptoms will either disappear at puberty or get worse.

Although the nature of allergy is unpredictable, a balance theory explains how allergies can be controlled. It is thought that exposure to several allergens around the same time can cause symptoms, even if each one of those allergens is usually mild and does not cause significant symptoms. For example, a boy has mild allergies to dust, mold, and dog dander. At home, dust and mold are very well controlled. He visits his grandparents, however, and they have a very old home with a musty odor and many items that produce dust. Even though his dog stays home, the boy has an asthma attack because his system is overwhelmed with this exposure.

2

FOOD ALLERGY

I t is not uncommon for infants to have food allergies. However, it may sometimes be difficult to determine whether an infant is having an allergic reaction to a food or a problem in the intestinal tract. Some babies' intestinal tracts are not fully developed until the age of one. Colic seen in a child older than three months might indicate a food allergy. Since the diet of small children changes as they grow, it becomes more and more complicated to determine what food is causing a particular allergy. By preschool age, a child is eating a large variety of foods.

Food allergies in children can cause ear, eye, and nose symptoms, hives, digestive problems, asthma, or eczema. Some children may have one or more of these allergy conditions.

Some babies constantly have irritated bottoms or rashes around their mouths. Other children suffer from digestive problems or eczema. It is possible for a child to develop a stuffy nose with one food and a skin rash with another. With food allergy, symptoms may be brief or may last several hours. In a severe reaction, an allergic child can go into shock.

A typical gastrointestinal allergy to a food might start with itching and possibly swelling around the mouth and lips. If there is no reaction until later, nausea, vomiting, and/or diarrhea may occur as a strong reaction. Milder reactions might include cramps, pain, loose stool, or hives.

Some recent research shows that certain preventive measures may delay or even be able to eliminate allergy in a child. A pregnant woman can change her diet and environment. She will need to avoid foods that commonly cause allergy and to eliminate as much as possible common household allergens. If she decides to nurse her baby, she will need to continue to avoid common food allergens. These measures are particularly wise when both parents have allergies.

Food allergies are difficult to diagnose because allergy skin tests are not reliable. When these tests show a positive reaction to a food, however, they can offer guidance for observation of symptoms. Further review with diet diaries and elimination diets are necessary to confirm a food allergy. How to conduct an elimination diet is discussed later.

Babies are not old enough to have built up IgE antibodies in their blood, and they usually test negative for food skin tests. If the child is nursing only, the mother may be eating something that upsets the child. For bottle-fed babies, physicians usually find it easier to switch formulas until symptoms cease.

When foods appear to cause significant allergy, only avoidance diets help. For some reason, antihistamines do not help gastrointestinal allergy, but relieve other symptoms caused by food allergy, such as hives. Food elimination diets and foods that seldom cause allergy are discussed in Key 46.

3

~~~~~~

HAY FEVER (ALLERGIC RHINITIS)

We all are familiar with the person who sneezes and complains of itching and watering of the eyes and nose. These are the most common symptoms of hay fever, or allergic rhinitis. Some people mistakenly think rhinitis is a cold or flu. However, allergic rhinitis does not last for a specific period of time, and it itches.

When children are too young to describe symptoms, the length of time that symptoms last becomes important. A cold usually starts with a sore throat and lasts about ten days. An allergy may cause a stuffy nose for a day or two, or for much longer than a cold.

There are several forms of rhinitis and an allergic child may have more than one. For example, the child may be allergic and have vasomotor rhinitis, a condition aggravated by irritants in the environment. And sometimes, when used in excess, nasal sprays cause rhinitis.

Allergic rhinitis can be caused by different allergens at different times of the year. For example, grasses, trees, and weeds pollinate at the same time each year. If a person has allergy symptoms every May, and only in May, olive tree pollen would be one of the suspected causes. Symptoms occurring at the same time each year could also result from seasonal food. If a person experiences allergic rhinitis symptoms year-round, the physician will most likely suspect an environmental allergy, with the possible culprit allergen being a family pet, house dust, or some other substance in the home.

Hay fever is a misleading term because it includes several symptoms of the upper airway. Since children may not communicate their discomforts, there are classical ways to recognize a youngster with allergy.

The "allergic salute" is common to children with allergy. Very young children do not know how to communicate itching or may not even be aware of the symptom. Almost as a reflex, they may push up the nose with a hand to relieve the itching. This is the allergic salute. This pushing maneuver temporarily opens the airway so they can breathe better. It is also not unusual to see allergic children making funny faces to relieve itching. They may wrinkle up their noses bunny-style or grimace for a second. Or they may twist their mouths from side to side.

In addition to these discomforts, allergic children may experience eye and ear symptoms. Their eyes and lids can become red, swollen, or itchy, and matter may run from them; this condition is called allergic conjunctivitis. These symptoms usually accompany other allergy reactions, but sometimes only eye symptoms appear.

The ear may feel full and hurt. Ears can present problems in infants and small children until the age of five. The eustachian tube that runs from the ear to the throat may swell and trap fluid. This occurs because the tube is almost horizontal in the small child. As the child grows, the tube assumes the normal downward position and functions much better.

Youngsters with constant allergy symptoms often lack energy for play and schoolwork, and may not be able to play and learn to their full capacity.

4

ASTHMA

Asthma affects almost 10 percent of the children in the United States. Many people do not realize that an asthma attack can be very serious, and even fatal. Asthma requires the diligence of the physician, the parents, and the child once he or she is old enough to assume this responsibility.

Asthma has recently been redefined. In the past, spasm or restriction of the airways was perceived as the problem. Now, it is defined as a combination of airway obstruction, inflammation, and increased responsiveness to air pollutants and allergies. Inflammation is playing a key role.

Frequently asthma is underdiagnosed, especially in small children, and is often mistaken for bronchitis or pneumonia. Allergens, viruses, and exercise can cause asthma.

The symptoms of asthma usually begin after the age of two; however, even small babies can have asthma. Some children suffer from both hay fever and asthma. Instead of the hay fever sufferer's nose being the affected area, the asthmatic's lungs respond to the allergens. Allergic children whose target area for allergic response is the bronchial airways and lungs get asthma. After the antibody attaches to an allergen and the chain of chemical reactions occur, inflammation results. This early phase of asthma begins within hours. In a later phase, the release of more chemicals swells and congests air passages even more.

7

Asthma attacks vary from child to child. Some experience instant breathing difficulty when exposed to an allergen or irritant. Some children get a tight chest only when they exercise. Others develop asthma at the end of a cold or flu.

Children may not recognize or know how to say that they have restricted breathing. A physician can quickly pick up with a stethoscope wheezing sounds that you cannot hear. If you can detect the wheezes without a stethoscope, the airways are 50 percent or more constricted. A child having a severe asthma attack may not have any sound in part of the lungs. Inflammation and mucus fill these areas so air cannot be exchanged.

A typical attack starts with a cough or a feeling of tightness in the chest. After a day, the inflamed linings of the airways swell to make breathing even more difficult. The type of medication and the speed with which it is administered can control the severity of the attack. Recent changes in the care of asthma enables physicians to prevent the condition from becoming as serious as it has been in the past.

Inhalers are small aerosol devices that can deliver many different combinations of medications. Some are used to prevent the antibody reaction; others work to open constricted bronchial airways. Daily medications given to asthmatics insure that the passages are kept open. Once an attack begins, there are medicines for both early and late phases.

There are four components in the treatment of asthma. The first is education of the parents and child. The second is environment. Changes that eliminate allergens in the environment are very important. Drug therapy to open airways and reduce inflammation at the right time is the critical third component. The fourth component is the daily monitoring of lung functions. Hand-held meters, called Peak Flow Meters, are used by parents and children to note changing functions. By catching an asthma attack in the warning stage when functions begin to drop, medication changes can head off an attack.

Recent advances in understanding this condition have resulted in new medicines to better control each phase of the asthma attack. Interest in the linings of the airways has focused research on the chemicals released there. New medications to combat the release of specific chemicals at certain stages of the attack will be designed.

Just a few years ago, very little was known about asthma, and there was considerable talk about the cause being psychological.

Children with asthma can suffer psychological damage because of the restriction of normal activities when they are ill. This can affect their social development, their progress in school, and their family life. It is important not to label a child as an asthmatic, a term indicating that the child has a special problem requiring care. Instead, teachers, friends, and parents must consider the well-being of the whole child and treat the asthma just as a condition of an otherwise healthy child.

5

~~~~~~

ECZEMA (ALLERGIC DERMATITIS)

E czema, or allergic dermatitis, is an irritation of the skin inflamed by scratching because of intense itching. Skin lesions result and weeping ensues.

The causes of eczema are unknown, but many children with eczema have been found to be allergic to such things as pollen or house dust. Eczema can begin during the first couple of months after birth. Inflamed red areas that may weep begin to appear, along with crusting on the face, scalp, or extremities. Inflamed areas eventually appear in the creases of the elbows and legs. This condition may subside around the age of three or four, although there may be occasional flare-ups during childhood or later in life. Some of these children will have hay fever or asthma as they grow older.

Before eczema was better understood, it was thought that someone with this skin disorder could not sweat. It is now known that dry skin is characteristic of the condition, but that the patient's skin actually perspires more than the normal person's. Because of the sweating, skin preparations need to be frequently reapplied.

Itching starts an itch-scratch-rash-itch cycle. The urge to rub or scratch is so strong that it is difficult to ignore. If the child does not scratch, the skin will be clear—an obvious conclusion to all but the victim! The skin of children who have had eczema for several years takes on a leathery appearance. The constant scratching causes a scarring that thickens the skin.

For a diagnosis of allergic dermatitis, several features must be present. There must be itching and a typical pattern of redness on the face and body. There must be a repeated tendency for the skin to clear and then become inflamed again. In addition, there is usually a family history of allergies. These children, as a rule, test positive in allergy skin tests.

There are several signs that a physician will look for by conducting a physical examination and blood tests. However, because of obvious skin irritation, allergy skin tests may risk further skin inflammation. Another test, RAST (radioallergosorbent), requiring only a blood sample, may be used instead.

With the diagnosis of eczema, the physician will provide detailed instructions on bathing, lubricating, and treating the skin as part of the child's everyday routine.

6

HIVES (URTICARIA AND ANGIOEDEMA)

I n some allergic children, only their skin will react. Urticaria, the medical term for hives, is a skin disorder accompanied by itching and swelling that is quite common in children. As with many skin conditions, the cause is difficult to determine. Children can get hives from viruses, illness, medications, foods, or other sources. The key to discovering the cause is the child's history. Several questions must be answered. Does the child have a fever or is he or she receiving antibiotics? If there is no illness, are the hives a result of a food allergy? Could the hives be the result of contact with an allergen such as grass or the family cat?

There are acute and chronic forms of urticaria. The acute form usually has an obvious cause; once identified, it can be avoided. Even if it doesn't have an obvious cause, a single episode of hives does not warrant an allergy workup. Most acute forms are limited and do not recur. The acute form usually lasts from two to three hours, but some cases have been known to last up to seven days.

With the chronic form of hives, it is difficult to find a cause. The chronic form occurs as often in nonallergic as in allergic people. Sometimes a medicine or chemical that is frequently taken can cause the skin eruption. Penicillin in milk, over-the-counter medicines, dyes, or other food additives are just a few of the potential causes of chronic hives.

Some undiagnosed diseases may first begin with urticaria as the only noticeable symptom.

Urticaria can occur from medications, food or food additives, blood transfusions, allergens, infection, insects, and many other sources. As in other allergic conditions, antihistamines, steroids, and avoidance are the main line of defense.

Angioedema is an allergy skin condition that manifests itself in a form similar to giant hives that cause swelling in the deeper layers of the skin. The hands, feet, eyelids, or lips can puff up out of proportion. Edema in the upper airways may produce breathing difficulties, with the result that this condition is sometimes mistaken for asthma.

Angioedema as an allergy condition is not as common as the ones already discussed and requires a physician to diagnose. It is not as obvious as hives and can mimic many illnesses. Sometimes angioedema is life-threatening—for example, when the throat swells, possibly cutting off respiration. Although angioedema is usually restricted to a particular area of the body, it can be just as life-threatening as anaphylaxis, which affects the whole body.

7

SHOCK (ANAPHYLAXIS)

This condition is life threatening and requires immediate care. Anaphylactic shock is a severe reaction that can follow ingestion of a particular food or a stinging insect. These are the two most common causes. This profound reaction is the result of an outpouring of chemicals by the body upon exposure to the allergen.

It takes at least one exposure to the allergen before the shock reaction occurs. It also takes one exposure to build up IgE antibody. Sometimes there is a warning during an exposure to one of these life-threatening allergens. For example, a child is stung by a bee. Hives or swelling begins immediately and goes beyond the site of the sting. Sometimes it may take several exposures to a bee sting before a severe reaction occurs. With each sting, a little more swelling occurs—if the sting is on the toe the first time, the toe, toes, or foot may swell. Later, when another bee stings near the ankle, the entire foot and the ankle may swell. The second sting may result in anaphylaxis.

Children who experience unusual swelling, hives, or other symptoms after a sting should be seen by an allergist as they may need to be tested for stinging insect allergy. If the test is positive, the parents and the school will be given a bee sting kit containing an injection of epinephrine to control the shock. This gives time to get the child to a physician for assessment and further treatment. Allergy shots may be necessary. (For further information on insect allergies, see Key 41.)

If a food causes the reaction, parents, other caretakers, and teachers will need to watch the diet of a young child. Foods known to have caused anaphylaxis include eggs and shellfish. Nuts (for example, peanuts, Brazil nuts, pistachios, and cashews), other types of seafood, and camomile tea have also caused this reaction.

In complicated cases of anaphylaxis, where the exposure is not obvious, a variety of substances can be responsible, including horse serum, hormones, enzymes, allergy extracts, diagnostic agents, vitamins, antibiotics, Novocaine, and drugs.

The reaction usually starts five to ten minutes after an exposure. There may be skin redness, itching, a general feeling of anxiety, nausea, vomiting, abdominal cramping, light-headedness, shortness of breath, or difficulty swallowing. You can recognize these symptoms because the child will first flush and then become pale. Later he or she will turn deep red or purple. The heart rate will speed up and the child will be anxious. Treatment begins with the emergency administration of epinephrine. Other support measures are then taken by paramedics or emergency services physicians.

A mild form of anaphylaxis will come on slowly—a delayed onset of general symptoms that are not at the site of a sting. These may include urticaria, asthma, or other complaints. At the time of a sting there may not be swelling. If the allergy is from food, there may not be mouth irritation at the time of ingestion. Because these symptoms are not dramatic like anaphylaxis, they can be thought of as a partial anaphylaxis, but they should not be ignored. A physician should evaluate these symptoms in case there is a future exposure that will cause a full anaphlaxis.

Special instructions are given to people with these life-threatening allergies on how to avoid exposures. Careful monitoring of the diet by parents and teachers is necessary until the child with a food allergy is old enough to take the responsibility. A child so sensitive to a food that it can cause shock, must be educated early about avoiding the allergy-causing food. This is especially difficult for some foods (eggs, for example, because eggs are used to give texture to many foods). Children must learn to ask about casseroles, mixed-food dishes, and packaged foods. Once they can read, children must be taught to read labels.

Special instructions for parents of children allergic to stinging insects include information on where bees may be found, what attracts them, and how to avoid stings. In general, life-threatening bee stings require allergy shots. Other potential sources for a shock reaction tend to be medically related medications or diagnostic dyes. In the medical or dental setting, trained personnel are prepared to respond to this potential emergency.

8

ALLERGIES CAN CHANGE

Allergies can change for different reasons. The climate may encourage more pollen one year and not the next. As a child enters puberty his or her allergies may get worse or better. Sometimes moving to another part of the country gives relief.

Since every allergic person has a specific cause for the condition, it is difficult to determine if a child will outgrow the allergies. In general, as children reach puberty they tend to have less difficulty with symptoms.

Although there are no ways to determine with certainty whether a child will get better or worse at puberty, children receiving allergy injections for a few years may have a better chance of reducing their allergies. Then, by the time they become teenagers, allergy will no longer be forcing lifestyle changes upon them. Usually, they can quit the allergy shots. At this point a teen may experience only short and mild episodes of symptoms during particular pollen seasons or exposures to allergens.

There is a common belief that, if you move, the allergies will disappear. This may or may not be true. Moving from Connecticut, for example, to Arizona may bring relief from symptoms for about two years. It takes about that much time to acquire the allergens of that area. Such an example was a military family that moved every two years to a new duty station. At their last assignment, they stayed six years. During the third year at the same location, three family members began to have allergy symptoms.

If the family moves, taking their pet cat with them, and the child appears to no longer have a cat allergy, it may be due to an extensive reduction in allergens. Because the child has no allergies to the pollens in the new area, the cat is no longer a problem. As the child becomes sensitized to these new pollens, however, the cat will again become a problem.

Another example of detecting why allergy symptoms disappear and reappear concerns a family that moved from the Midwest to the Arizona/Nevada border. Their furnishings were ideally suited to prevent allergy problems. Upon arrival in Arizona, they stored the furniture in a garage. After six months, they found a new home. After moving into it, their two children started having symptoms. The parents finally realized that so much dust had collected while their furniture was in storage that they had created an allergy source. Fortunately, they could have everything cleaned.

9

WEATHER AND AIR POLLUTION

The weather gets blamed for so many problems and allergy is one of them. Weather conditions that produce winds often stir up pollens that have settled. The dust that blows may or may not contain pollens that cause allergy symptoms. These winds can also irritate the respiratory tract so that allergy symptoms are more likely.

On the West Coast there is a wind condition called Chinook in the Northwest and Santa Ana in the Southwest. With these winds, the air becomes very dry. As a result, the respiratory tract becomes irritated from lack of moisture. These strong winds stir up pollens and dust to further irritate allergic people. It is not unusual for a large percentage of allergic people to have headaches as the high-pressure air moves into their area.

Areas of the country that are along large lakes or coasts tend to be high in humidity. Warm air and high humidity encourage the growth of molds. There are actually mold seasons just like pollen seasons in some of these areas. In very damp climates, mold growth inside homes becomes a problem for children allergic to these organisms. The house dust mites also thrive in these climates.

In areas where there is a constant warm, humid climate, the pollen and mold seasons may last year-round. For example, the southern California coastal climate really has no winter. There are grasses, weeds, and trees blooming all year.

The areas that have distinct seasons have a break from pollens once the first frost in the fall has come until spring. Depending upon the area and altitude, some locations may have excessive pollens in the air. These pollens might include ragweed, which grows so profusely that some communities actually organize parties to rid the area so their families will suffer less.

In many of our major cities, air pollution is the cause of several debilitating physical symptoms. For children who already have compromised breathing, air pollution is a major irritant. Each city's pollutants are unique to it, depending upon its industry and other sources for pollutants. The quality of the air of every city needs to be investigated. Even a small town could have a problem if a particular industry is located near it. Cities that do monitor air quality usually issue staged alerts through the media to warn people with respiratory problems to stay indoors. In addition, health professionals will offer suggestions on when to exercise or play outdoors.

As a rule, air quality in the larger cities is worse later in the week than on the weekend and in the beginning of the week. Air quality is better during the weekend, during rain, and under certain wind conditions, and it is better early in the morning than it is later in the day. The warm, humid, still, and sunny days of summer make air quality worse.

10

~~~~~~

PREPARING YOUR CHILD TO VISIT THE ALLERGIST

If your pediatrician or family physician has made a referral to the allergist, prepare your child for the visit. Explain to a preschooler or older child what is going to happen. Children have often heard scary stories about getting hundreds of shots in their back. By learning about the process of the workup and the reasons for having it, children can approach it as something positive to accomplish rather than as a negative experience that causes fear and anxiety.

Tell your child that you will first talk to the doctor, who will ask questions about the child's symptoms. With an older child, you can discuss what you think is causing symptoms or where the youngster is when symptoms occur. Write down the answers so your child gets involved in the process. Your child might even take this list to the doctor as a reminder. With a younger child, you need only mention that you are going to talk to the doctor about the child's stuffy nose or some other symptom.

Explain that, after you talk, the doctor will give the child a physical examination, during which the physician will look in the ears, nose, and mouth to see if there is swelling or soreness. The doctor will also listen with a stethoscope to hear how she or he breathes. Show the child a picture of a stethoscope if you have one.

After finishing the examination, the doctor will probably order some tests. Children with asthma should be told that they will take some breathing tests. Tell them they may have to blow into a machine so the doctor or technician can see how they breathe. Sometimes the doctor will ask a child to blow into a hand-held meter.

Tell your child what will happen during the skin tests. The technician will draw on the child's arm or back to make a map of spots that are to be tested. Explain that a little needlelike stick will press into the skin after a drop of fluid has been put on it. There will be a slight prick feeling but it will not hurt very much. In a few minutes some of these prick spots will itch, but the itch will go away after a while. The technician will measure each spot. If your child is of elementary school age, you might want to go into more detail, depending upon the questions being asked. With a younger child, however, wait until you are at the doctor's office. Ask the technician what will occur next and then explain it to your child.

When the skin tests are finished, the doctor may want a few intradermal tests. These will be done with a syringe. The needle puts a bubble of fluid under the skin. This feels like the skin test prick but lasts just a little bit longer. After a few minutes these spots will also itch. The technician will again measure the itching spots.

Characteristically, there is a weltlike eruption (called a wheal) with redness around it. Both the wheal and the red area are measured, and the size of these wheals is compared with two or three spots called controls. The control is a re-active spot purposely given to see how much the skin has the capacity to react. The technician will explain if your child is asking more questions. After the skin tests, the doctor will talk to you.

If your child is too young for you to explain what will happen in the allergist's office, there are a couple of things you can do to calm the child's fears. One is to insist that you hold the child facing you during the skin tests. The technician easily can work on the back, and your child has the comfort of the parent.

Usually the parent can be present during skin tests. As a rule, parents add comfort and assurance. Sometimes, how-ever, young and immature parents are not at ease with this testing. If the child is aware of their uneasiness, he or she may not remain still enough to undergo the tests. The tech-nician may ask the parents to leave the room and return in a few minutes.

Depending upon how much allergies are affecting the child's normal life, the physician will probably advise you to make some changes. You will discuss how to fix your child's bedroom to avoid allergens.

In addition, the doctor may decide that allergy shots would be of benefit. At this point, it is good to take your child to the shot room, so that the youngster can see what happens and will know what to expect. Have the technician select a willing child to demonstrate the ease of getting a shot, so that your child can see exactly what is going to happen. Most children are quite proud of themselves when getting these shots if they behave well.

The children who scream and cry when they have shots are usually unprepared. For some good reason, known to the parent and physician, they are going to have something done to them but they do not know what it is. They are terrified. On the other hand, those who know what to expect are usually matter-of-fact when telling their friends about the visit to the doctor.

Depending on the age of your child, the allergy workup may require more than one visit. If this is the case, ask the nurse or doctor to describe what will happen on the next visit. It would not be unusual for X rays, laboratory, or other diagnostic tests to be requested.

Once the workup is complete, emphasize how well your child behaved. If the visit was difficult, point out what *did* go well and tell your child that you are proud. Because the relationship with the allergist is ongoing, it is important to keep the sessions as positive as possible.

11

~~~~~~

SKIN TESTS AND WHAT THEY MEAN

A s medical science continues to improve methods of treating allergies, we will see future changes in testing and medications. There are a few ways that the American Academy of Allergy and Immunology recognizes for testing for allergies.

One is the traditional skin test described in Key 10. Under some circumstances, another test—radioallergosorbent test (RAST)—is offered. Using a blood sample from the patient, the test measures the IgE antibody in the blood serum for each allergen. This test is good for small children or children with sensitive skin.

Some other tests, not recognized by the Academy, should be avoided. They include cytotoxicity testing (Bryan's test), urine autoinjection (autogenous urine immunization), and provocative and neutralization testing. Contact the Academy for further information.

Although most allergists will test for common foods that cause allergy, be aware that skin tests are not conclusive. The only sure way to determine a food allergy is through avoidance diets and challenge testing. For this reason, skin testing for foods is usually limited to about ten foods. However, since foods play an important part in early life, the physician will probably want to test for a food allergy. The RAST appears to be more reliable for food testing. (See Key 46 for more information.)

When the skin tests are complete, your physician will most likely share the results with you. The skin test sheet usually has a list of Latin names followed by the common names. The technician's measurements will guide the allergist's opinions as to what the significant allergies are. It is important that you understand each of the positive tests so that you can look for and identify these substances in the environment.

It is common to include the trees, grasses, and weeds in allergy shots because they cannot be eliminated from the environment. However, you need to learn to identify them so they can be avoided under certain circumstances. For example, if the tests show that your child has a strong allergy to elm trees, your concern is to recognize, learn about, and try to avoid these trees. When they are pollinating, you would not picnic with your youngster in a park with elm trees. Or, if elms grow on the street where you live, you would probably have to keep the home closed and filtered during the pollination season. Your child can play either inside or in an outside area free of elms until the pollination season is over. Gradually, the use of allergy shots will make these measures less necessary.

Depending upon the area in which you live, molds can be seasonal just like pollens. However, molds are also prevalent in damp areas in the home. In Key 25, there are guidelines on how to eliminate them.

Environmental allergens listed on the skin test sheet will include house dust, dust mites, pets, animal and plant fibers, and a few others. Animal and plant fibers include wool, kapok, cottonseed, and flax.

12

~~~~~~

YOU AND YOUR CHILD ARE ON THE HEALTHCARE TEAM

Allergy is one area of medicine where good results depend upon teamwork. Responsibility for health improvement belongs to you, the doctor, and your child if she or he is old enough to handle new responsibilities. The physician's part is to determine what is causing trouble and provide a treatment plan. The physician should also provide information about allergens and about ways in which you can provide a good environment for your child. Your part is to determine where the allergens are and to assist your child in learning to take responsibility for her health. This includes taking medicines properly and learning how to adjust her lifestyle to avoid symptoms.

Once the child is old enough, your role will be to monitor that responsibility. If all the team members play their part, there should be no hospitalizations or severe allergy attacks. Allergists, who create a care team, pride themselves on the fact that they have low admitting rates to hospitals. In fact, some even lose privileges at the local hospital because they do not admit enough patients.

If your child has to be admitted several times, look for a lack of understanding by one of the team members—good

27

communication is essential. An exception might be a child with severe asthma. Keep in mind, however, that repeated hospitalizing does not mean that, as a parent, you are failing in some way. Some asthmatics are ill for physical reasons that can be very difficult to control. Your allergist or pulmonologist will be happy to explain the reasons and discuss the circumstance with you.

Most allergists have trained their staffs to handle all manner of questions. If you find it difficult to talk to the doctor when you are worried, call and speak to the nurse. Nurses field questions and also know when the doctor needs to participate. If you have questions about your child's shots, call the nurse or the medical assistant who gives the shots. The important thing, when in doubt, is to ask about what to do. This strengthens the team communication.

13

~~~

THE TRIGGERS FOR ALLERGY SYMPTOMS

There are several categories of allergens, including inhalants, ingestants, injectants, contactants, and infectants. Inhalants are the most common sources for allergy symptoms.

Inhalant. Particles that we breathe, such as dust, vapors, animal danders, feathers, or inhaled medications, can cause allergy.

Ingestants. Another category is ingestants, anything we eat or drink, including beverages, medicines, and vitamins. See Key 46 for more information.

Injectants. Injectants can enter the body in one of two ways. One is through an insect sting. The other is through needle injection that would include a medication. See Keys 41, 42, and 43.

Contactants. Allergic skin reactions can occur when some substance comes into contact with the skin. Some clothing, metals, leather, and other items can cause a contact allergy. Contact with pollen grains or grass while playing can cause a hive, which is an IgE antibody reaction. The hive is, in effect, a mini skin test.

Infectants. Some organisms have an allergic effect on the body whether or not there is an infection. These might include bacteria, fungi (mold), or parasites. This book covers only common allergies related to the IgE antibody. Sometimes, IgE antibody reactions are referred to as *immediate hypersensitivity.*

Inhalants include pollens, molds, and environmentals. Pollens exist everywhere and are active during certain seasons. For example, grasses mostly pollinate during the spring, trees during the early summer, and weeds during the late summer and early fall.

The pollens that cause allergy are wind-borne. They are very light so the wind can carry them over great distances. The plants that are wind-pollinated occur in temperate regions such as the United States and Canada. In countries near the equator, the humidity makes the pollen too heavy to be wind-borne. As a result, showy plants in these areas depend upon insects and bees to pollinate them.

Plants must have certain characteristics to be an allergen. They must be seed-bearing such as evergreens and some flowering plants. They must also produce a large amount of pollen and grow over wide areas. Mosses or ferns, which produce spores that drop on the ground or are carried by animals, do not have the characteristics needed to be an allergen.

Molds are also a major player in allergies. Molds can be found indoors and outdoors and are difficult to remove from the environment.

Some molds are seasonal, such as pollens. These molds are prevalent in seasonal crops or foliage. Fall leaves, for example, are notorious for producing mold allergy. It is the action of molds that eventually breaks down the leaves to form mulch.

Some molds are seasonal because the climate is good for them at a certain time. The humidity and warm temperature provide the environment they need to reproduce. States that border large bodies of water may have mold seasons in late summer or fall.

Molds are apparent in everyday life. The darkening of the grout in between bath or kitchen tiles, the mildew on the shower curtain, or the mildew from the clothes hamper are common sources in the environment. Some foods, such as blue cheese, depend upon mold for flavor, while others that develop mold after a few days must be discarded. Not all molds cause allergy.

Besides pollens and molds, there are environmental allergens that cause allergy. These include plant or animal substances or products from them, such as house dust. Dust mites and pet dander are examples of allergens that may be part of house dust.

Also classified with these environmentals are air pollutants. Chemicals in the air are irritants rather than allergens. They trigger allergy symptoms and upset the balance in the control of allergies. Other triggers for allergy include your child's lifestyle and emotions.

14

A QUESTION OF BALANCE

With one or more allergic members in a family, a healthy and happy lifestyle becomes a challenge. Years ago, physicians provided strict rules for allergy environment control, and for the child's play and diet. Today, in evolving a treatment plan, most physicians will try to balance treatment goals and treatment options.

The balancing is a good example of the art of medicine. The physician will evaluate your financial capability to support medicine, allergy shots, changes in the home, and other factors. For example, sometimes the parents are very young and overwhelmed. Sometimes both parents work and resort to caregivers to be with their child. These situations and the seriousness of your child's allergy problem will also go into the formula for the treatment plan. Your commitment to the treatment program is important.

If your child is missing school, lagging in social development, or doing poorly in school, the treatment plan will be more aggressive. The allergist will determine what medicines will be best for your child's particular circumstances.

Sometimes a child's allergy condition is mild. To prevent the condition from getting worse, many physicians elect initially to provide minimal medication and to rely on the parents to make some environmental changes. If the child is not better in a couple of months, allergy shots, an elimination diet, or diferent medication are some of the other alternatives.

Balance

Allergic Person In Balance

Allergic Person Out of Balance

Reprinted from the *Allergy Environment Guidebook,*
© 1989 by J. Bachman, Ph.D.

15

ACHIEVING BALANCE—
THE ROLE OF
ALLERGY SHOTS

I f pollens and molds represent a major portion of your
child's allergies, most allergists will begin with allergy
shots. Most likely, medicines will keep the symptoms
under control until the shots work. It may take more than a
year for the shots to build up to a level that alleviates symptoms.

At first, the dosage in the allergy shot is very weak. Your
child may go once or twice a week. As the dosage strength
increases, the visits will drop to one a week. By the time your
child is at the top strength, the office visits will be about every
three weeks. This is considered the maintenance dose. Most
children stay on the shots for two to four years at this level,
and then stop the injections.

Under some conditions, the shots must be cut back. For
example, the dosage level may be too high during a particular
pollen season, or your child may get the flu or some other
illness that requires missing an injection. If your child has a
small redness and swelling around the injection site, don't be
alarmed—this is not unusual. However, if noticeable swelling
continues, with an increase of symptoms or fatigue, tell the
physician. He or she can evaluate if the shots should be
changed.

In order to balance the strength of each allergy shot, the allergist will mix dilutions of those allergens to which your child may have strong reactions. Sometimes the bottles will be mixed so that all the pollens are in one bottle. When the pollens are in season, that solution can be given in weaker doses until the pollination is no longer occurring. It is not unusual for some children to start allergy shots with three vials, but once they reach a maintenance level, they may need only one.

It may be difficult to determine just what dosage to give during times of stress, illness, or pollen seasons. Slight adjustments can help control discomfort. Sometimes, the physician may adjust medications rather than the shots; otherwise, your child will never reach the top maintenance level.

When the treatment plan is started, keep in mind that it is not permanent. New medications, changes in the environment, or an illness may alter the program. You should not be disturbed if the doctor makes changes. A flexible treatment plan needs to accommodate all of the changes in a growing child's life.

16

~~~~~~

ACHIEVING BALANCE— THE ROLE OF MEDICINE

There are many combinations of medicines for the treatment of allergies and many different varieties on the market, including medicines for prevention, control, maintenance, and emergencies.

For allergic rhinitis, or hay fever, decongestants and antihistamines are still the favored medications. Besides the antihistamines and decongestants, there are steroid nasal sprays, nasal Cromolyn, and oral steroids. Steroids are considered the big guns, reserved for special circumstances. Cromolyn, discussed later, helps prevent symptoms. Sleepiness has been a major side effect of antihistamines, but there are now medications that do not cause drowsiness. In general, children with rhinitis require very little medication.

Asthma sufferers have a long list of medications to control spasm and inflammation. Some drugs serve to prevent symptoms, others to control them during different phases of an attack. Medication dosage and type are guided but depend upon readings on the Peak Flow Meter. This hand-held device measures lung functioning These medications are the most important factors in controlling asthma, while most other allergic conditions, are not major components in treatment. Medicines used in asthma are variations of three classes of drugs.

Adrenergic medications, known as beta-adrenergic, beta agonist, or adrenaline-type medications, help to dilate the air passages to the lungs. Adrenalin, used less today because of new drugs, has long been the mainstay in emergency rooms. Its immediate dilation effect on the airways is still occasionally required. Side effects include anxiety, shakiness, headache, and an irregular or pounding heartbeat. Because of this profound effect, physicians now use a lower dose in a mist or nebulizer that goes deep into the lungs. The side effects are minimal. Children who suffer asthma attacks that require an emergency visit to the doctor or hospital can now have a nebulizer in the home.

Metered inhalers are very important for special situations. These pocket-size aerosol devices can be kept in the nurse's office at school. Older children can carry them with them. Inhalers may contain albuterol (the generic name for the brands Proventil and Ventolin), metaproterenol (brand names Alupent or Metaprel), or terbutaline (brand names Brethaire and Brethine).

Inhalers require careful training for proper use. They are used under certain circumstances for specific levels of the asthma attack. If a child gets asthma from exercise or cold air, the inhaler can be used in advance to prevent a problem from developing. It can also be used to open airways before other medications to be sure of adequate dosage. Your physician will advise you when and how these medications should be used.

Obviously, if you have a very young child with asthma, other medication options are considered, including oral forms of asthma medications. The side effects of these oral forms are a problem in small children. They may be too young to complain about stomach pain or they may vomit the medication so the amount of the dosage is not known. Physicians

37

do not agree on the best solution. Some believe that there is a positive effect even if the dosage is below the side-effect level. Because each child is unique and each physician has had different experience, it is best to discuss this. There may be other alternatives.

Theophylline has been a mainstay medication for asthma. Recently, some new medications have begun to replace it. Used daily, theophylline serves as a preventive medication by maintaining open airways. Unfortunately, to reach the blood levels needed to control asthma, there are side effects. Some children become overactive or get an upset stomach and headache. For these children, there are many brands to choose from. Different brands offer different combination of drugs to combat the side effects.

Steroids (corticosteroids) are very valuable in the treatment of asthma. They decrease the resulting inflammation that occurs in the lung passageway and reduce mucus production from the lining of the airways. They also calm the tendency for the airways to react. This calming enables other medications to work better. Most important, they prevent the formation of chemicals that cause the bronchoconstriction. These medications can be delivered to the lungs by aerosol sprays. Some are packaged under the generic names of prednisone, prednisolone, and methylprednisolone.

Over the years, the side effects of steroids have been reduced. Today these medications are used orally for short periods of time or on special treatment schedules to avoid side effects. Used correctly, they are safe. If they are prescribed improperly for long periods of time, they can cause a number of problems, including increased appetite, a masked feeling of well-being, fluid retention, and weight gain. If children must take these medications, an allergist or pulmonologist should manage their care.

Cromolyn is an aerosol that serves as a preventive medication. Taken daily, it can block the release of chemicals that cause the asthma or a hay fever reaction. It is very safe for children; however, it is not as effective once an allergy attack has started. This medication is particularly good for asthma that is the result of exercise or for occasional exposures to allergens. When taken before the exposure, it can prevent symptoms.

The asthmatic child gets infections rather easily because of the inability to move secretions and air. Antibiotics are the drug of choice. Expectorants, used for years, have been found to be ineffective for asthma treatment.

Avoidance is the ideal element in achieving balance. It makes sense to remove an allergen when possible from the environment. Paying close attention to and eliminating some of the causes of allergy can help to reduce symptoms. Pollens, some molds, air pollution, and weather are beyond your control; however, eliminating a feather pillow or an old wool rug is not.

In general, food allergy requires avoidance. Some medicines will give symptom relief until the offending food is determined. Your doctor can suggest over-the-counter remedies to use for headache, stomachache, diarrhea, and other symptoms.

Children with eczema have routines for skin care that become part of every day. These include moisturizers for the skin, anti-itch creams or medicine, and protection of the skin from irritants. Children with highly sensitive skin need to cover it to prevent contact with pollens and materials to which they may be allergic.

17

ACHIEVING BALANCE— THE ROLE OF FEELINGS

As mentioned earlier, more than one family member may have allergies. The inherited tendency can result in allergies in one or more of the family members. If this is the case, it is really best to have one physician treating the family. In this way, the treatment plan becomes a family matter. Again, whether it is one child, several children, or the whole family, the focus should remain on the whole child or the whole family. Once allergy is singled out as a problem, an unhealthy focus can take place.

There is no reason that allergic children cannot participate in activities with their peers. Overprotecting can cause psychological problems for the family. Sometimes a mother becomes so focused on the allergic child and so overprotective that the child's life becomes quite restricted. In this case, the whole family suffers: the allergic child feels smothered, and the other family members feel resentment toward the allergic child. The balance of interactions among wife, husband, and children is affected.

When a child's allergy becomes the family focus, the marriage and the siblings do not receive the attention they require for healthy relationships. For example, take the case of a teenage daughter with severe asthma. An environmental study was conducted to see if an allergen exposure had been missed. The home had excellent environmental control. All the focus of daily living was on the asthmatic teenager. By overfocusing on their teen, the parents began to neglect their marriage and no longer had good communication with each other. The girl's illness had become the center of attention of the family. It is quite a responsibility to realize that if you get well, your parents will separate! In this case the whole family began counseling to improve their communication, and the daughter's asthma improved.

In another example, a five-year-old boy was adopted by a family with two daughters. He came to the home with severe asthma and behavior problems. The family believed that if they loved the boy, all would be well. Pretty soon the child commanded all the parents' attention, and the other two children were not getting their needs met. One daughter began to act out in school, the other daughter became withdrawn and isolated. Both started to do poorly in school. It took the social worker, physicians, and therapists to help the family through a difficult time.

It is easy to become overfocused on an asthmatic child because an attack is very frightening. A feeling of helplessness occurs when you see your child gasping for air. The youngster may get anxious because he or she feels as if the air supply is being cut off. Of course, you need to focus fully on your child when an attack occurs; however, by learning all you can about asthma, you can will be able to react calmly. As you learn more, you will find ways to help your child avoid attacks.

When it is discovered that the focus of family relationships is on the allergic child, there are options to deal with this situation. A few sessions with a family therapist can help to reestablish healthy relationships. One or more family members may require additional sessions, depending upon how long the problems have been going on. Maybe some help with housework will allow the parent or parents more quality time with siblings. Perhaps a knowledgeable caregiver for the asthmatic child or children will create time for the parents to enjoy each other.

Sometimes you or your other children may begin to resent the attention and time that the allergic child receives. You may find that your energy is low or that you feel angry because you are missing an activity you enjoy.

It is important to discuss any feelings that you or your children experience. If you don't pay attention to negative feelings, they can become problems. For example, you may be a single parent working full-time with active children who both suffer from allergies. You must drive them to school and activities, manage different schedules to accommodate the activities, and attend school functions. All this must be fitted into a schedule along with visits to the doctor, your usual housework, and religious activities. No doubt, you feel some resentment because you have a lot to do and very little time for yourself. You will need to become creative for alternatives to alleviate the stress. You might share driving or activity attendance with another parent so that you have less burden. You might attend a parents' group for allergic children, where you can share some of your difficulties and learn how other parents cope.

Check with the local Asthma and Allergy Foundation of America or the American Lung Association for parent support groups. In addition, some cities have their own parent support groups. Your allergist will know about them. Finding other people who are encountering the same negative feelings allows you to talk over the problems and get ideas on how you can better handle them. Typically, parents worry about the medications, time out from activities, and long-term effects their children may experience. These groups educate and support.

The total group has many individual experiences that can be shared. For example, if your grade-school-age child is ignoring symptoms and not telling his caregiver about them, the group will probably have suggestions that will help you and your child. It is also good to hear from others with the same experience that although you try to do everything right, your child still has problems. Someone in the group will be sure to support you, and reassure you that you are doing a good job.

18

INFANTS AND ALLERGY

Food allergy (see Key 46), is the most common cause of allergic symptoms in the small child. Since it takes up to two years to acquire an allergy to pollens, babies may not experience pollen allergy until a second season. Babies with allergic rhinitis or asthma from pollen are unusual; however, they may acquire similar symptoms from year-round exposure to pets, such as a cat or dog.

Since infants cannot tell you that they are having symptoms, allergy can easily go unrecognized. The most common causes of allergies in infants are cereals and milk. Babies can express allergy symptoms in different ways.

Gastrointestinal symptoms may include colic. Babies with colic will pull up their legs and scream with discomfort. As a rule, the baby experiencing colic after three months of age is suspect for an allergy. Some act hungry all the time. They have excess gas, spitting up, and diarrhea. It is wise to work with the physician to change formulas and introduce the foods that are least likely to cause symptoms of allergy.

Skin conditions including rash or eczema usually begin on the cheeks as bright red spots. The baby may also have a red bottom. Later, redness may appear in the creases of the arms and legs. On occasion, this inflammation can spread to cover the greater part of the child's body.

Children who are destined to have severe asthma frequently begin at a very young age with symptoms. You may observe the first signs when your baby wheezes or coughs while asleep. If the tummy is sucked in while breathing, your baby is putting more than usual effort into breathing. Sometimes you can see that the ribs and the area below the Adam's apple are sucked in as well. If you observe labored breathing, a chest rattle, or a wheeze, call your physician as soon as possible. It is important to attend to these conditions immediately, because the symptoms may get worse. If this should happen during the middle of the night, your physician may instruct you to go to an urgent care center or the hospital emergency room. The doctor who sees your baby there can decide if this is asthma or some other chest condition common to infants.

The stuffy nose with or without a watery mucus discharge may be the first signs of hay fever or allergic rhinitis. Frequently, the mother will notice that her baby is having difficulty nursing or taking formula. This may indicate that your baby can't breathe and eat at the same time. Parents will frequently complain that the baby has a cold all the time, but small babies with colds are unusual. The parents have to observe closely for symptoms of fever, and for thickened and/or colored nasal discharge that may represent an infection. In addition, the length of time of these colds will be important information that the doctor will ask for.

Some babies exhibit their allergies by being irritable. It is their way of communicating that something is not right. This irritability may also accompany a frequent need for sleep.

If there is a family history of allergies, pay special attention when introducing foods to the baby's diet. Since foods are the most common causes for allergies in infants, discuss with your physician when to introduce cow's milk or wheat or other cereals. Eggs, chicken, or products that include any of these ingredients should not begin until after the first year. At that time, introduce these foods one at a time at two-week intervals. Although the reason is not well understood, avoidance of these common allergenic foods early in life may eliminate the food allergy altogether. See Key 46 for more information.

The National Jewish Center for Immunology and Respiratory Medicine recently published a study linking parent behavior and subsequent development of asthma. The families studied had children at risk for asthma from family history. The study found that the primary caregiver's ability to cope during the child's first three years was a key to the probability of the child's having asthma in the future.

Dr. Mary Klinnert, a researcher on the study, indicated that evidence of early parenting difficulties can predict asthma. If a parent does not have coping skills, then counseling and stress reduction support programs may help decrease the incidence of asthma. This research should not suggest that asthma is caused by inadequate parenting.

19

PRESCHOOLERS AND
ALLERGY

I f your child is allergic, the preschool years are the time
when symptoms usually begin. It can be a very frustrating
time because the child is also beginning to socialize and
there are unavoidable exposures to childhood illnesses. Some
of these children are sick more often than their peers. Gradually they begin to show some of the signs that identify them
as an allergic child. Some exhibit a cranky behavior and lack
energy while others will have obvious symptoms of asthma
or hay fever.

Food allergies can still play an important part with these
young children. It becomes complicated to determine the
cause when there are pollen and environmental allergies as
well.

Your allergic child may be falling behind in social development because of not feeling well. If your child seems to
be ill more days than you believe is normal, it is worth consulting with an allergist to see how you can prevent the allergy
from getting worse. It is wise to get an opinion before the
school year begins so the child can enjoy school and do well.
Minimizing the allergy at this age will lessen complications
later. Let the doctor decide if your child needs attention now
or later.

Even though the preschool child is too young to take
responsibility for his or her care, there are several things that
can be done. You can lay the foundation for responsibility

later. First, you will want to learn as much about the condition as possible. This includes learning how the lungs work. If you know how they work normally, you can begin to recognize the onset of allergy symptoms and what the triggers may be. Next start to relay your observations to your child so that he learns to recognize early signs of an asthma attack. Gradually, you will notice he can understand when you explain in very simple terms what is happening in the body.

When your child starts telling you he needs medicine, you will know that you are ready for the next learning stage. Children will give you the necessary guidance on how much detail they need by their questions. Answer their many questions with simple, short statements. Sometimes they will ask the same question over and over until they fully understand the answer.

As you learn to eliminate or control the triggers or sources for allergy symptoms, you can point them out to your child. He or she will begin to connect symptoms with a cause later. During these early years, getting the child in touch with the onset of symptoms is about all you can expect. The cause-and-effect relationship will not be understood or, at most, it will not mean too much until the elementary school years.

You can balance your child's exposures, need for rest, and level of activity in concert with medications and other treatments the physician may have prescribed. Your child is too young to understand these concepts of balance until about age five. At that time you can start to verbalize what you are doing, and he will be able to make the connections more quickly.

Education brings confidence in your decision-making and reduces worry. Once your child approaches the elementary school years, you may observe an increased concern for health problems. If he is aware enough to worry, it is time to teach more about allergy. He also will have more confidence by being better informed. It is important to introduce new facts slowly to avoid overwhelming the youngster.

By the time your child enters school, he or she will be able to recognize warning symptoms and alert the teacher. Provide the teacher with guidelines regarding when you or the school nurse should be contacted.

Most children in this age group are prone to infections, as they become more social and are around more and more people. These illnesses (in addition to allergies) may result in an unusual amount of time away from normal activities. As long as your child's development milestones are met and learning skills for school are beginning to develop, you should not worry. However, never be reluctant to talk to your pediatrician about concerns that you may have.

20

~~~~~~

THE ELEMENTARY
SCHOOL YEARS

Normal children are quite social beings by the time they enter school. They have been taking responsibility for some of their own care for some time. They are now ready to take some responsibility for control of their health condition.

School-age children are beginning to understand their allergies. At this point, you can start to explain more about what is happening when allergy symptoms occur. By third grade, children are able to understand how the lungs work normally. They can recognize what medicine may be needed and why, and are ready to assume more responsibility for their health. Under your careful supervision, your child can now learn to make decisions about medicines.

One way to help children take responsibility for their medicines is to color code the bottles. Your doctor can assist you in labeling the drugs. If you start this practice in first grade, they will learn to associate the medicines with the different stages of their condition. For example, a daily medicine to prevent, maintain, or control symptoms may have a green sticker. A yellow sticker is on medicines to take when symptoms are increasing. A red-labeled medicine is for severe symptoms. Using the traffic light symbol, with its "Go" for green, "Caution" for yellow, and "Stop" for red, illustrates the stages in a way children can understand. Each time you give a medicine, be sure to emphasize the applicable stage of their condition. You should also discuss the need for restrictions in food or activity as the child moves from stage to stage.

Once children understand the colors and stages, start to name the medicine they are taking. Around the age of nine, they should be able to take the "green" medicine at a certain time each day on their own. By this time, they should also know the name of every medicine they take. Gradually, with guidance from you, they will learn when to take the "yellow" medicine and, if needed, change or restrict their activities.

Children will probably not be ready to decide when to take the "red" medicine until the end of sixth grade. By then they should know not only the brand names but the dosages they are taking.

The system just described teaches the child to assume some responsibility for and to make some decisions about his health. It also enlists him as a member of his own healthcare team. A child who is not part of the decision system will not assume the responsibility on his own. From the first day you see the doctor, involve your child in the decision-making.

The Asthma and Allergy Foundation of America and the American Lung Association, as well as local hospitals, offer a variety of programs. These organizations can direct parents to sources for teaching children about their allergies and asthma.

The Asthma and Allergy Foundation of America, in Los Angeles, offers an excellent program called ACT that uses the traffic light colors to teach decision-making. Some local lung associations offer programs for children with asthma.

Most children in second grade can start to make decisions about activity level and need for rest. It is important that they do not restrict activity as an excuse to get out of it or for the special attention they receive. Encourage your child to participate in all the social and learning activities.

Learning about health responsibilities can be extended to include learning about other responsibilities. There is no reason a child with allergies should not perform some chores. How to clean yet avoid allergy symptoms, for example, is part of learning about self-responsibility. However, there are two important "don'ts" on this chore list: one is vacuuming, the other is lawn mowing. If you do not have a central vacuum system and your child is sensitive to dust, she should be excused from this task. Wearing a mask is not appropriate when the allergen exposure can be avoided. For example, a child allergic to grass should not mow the lawn and, in fact, should not even be outside during mowing.

Teach your child about household repairs, or remodeling and redecorating the home. These useful experiences can reveal sources for allergies and enable you to discuss with the youngster how to eliminate or change them. Allergic children need also to be taught about the dangers to them inherent in certain cleaning products, aerosols, and furniture conditioners.

By age ten most children leave home for overnights and camp. The American Lung Association and the Asthma and Allergy Foundation offer special camps for children with moderate to severe asthma. Sleep-away camping gives children confidence to begin their lives as fully independent persons and is an important developmental step to independence.

21

TEEN TIMES

M any teenagers are capable of taking full responsibility for their health. The transition from monitoring your children to their assuming full responsibility usually begins around age thirteen. Eventually your role will be to observe how they are doing and have occasional discussions about their health. Talks should include setting goals for activities and offers of support to help them meet these goals. It is especially important to support your child when goals cannot be met because of illness. Such support should carry the message that setbacks like these are part of life—and not unusual at all. Work with your child to set flexible goals that allow for time out.

Once children have reached late grade school or the teen years, you should start talking about their readiness to handle their own health care. Indicate your confidence in them to handle their care themselves. You can further facilitate independence by encouraging a child to see the physician alone. Obviously, you will still be driving your teen to the doctor but you can remain in the waiting room. Then in the future you may wish to ask your teen if you can talk to the doctor. If you are uneasy about this, however, ask if you can all talk at the end of an office visit.

Because teenagers are beginning to assert their independence, peer activities become very important. Part of your support will be to make certain their activities maintain good health values. An asthmatic child experimenting with smoking or drugs can spell trouble. Help to supervise programs through school, church, or community.

The adolescent has by now become familiar with medications and with causes or triggers of allergy symptoms. Some youngsters are very conscientious and take full responsibility for their health. Other teens become anti-everything—most of all, of parents advising them what to do. Negotiate with your teen how he or she can communicate with you so that you are both comfortable.

One example of a successful agreement was that between a teenage son and his parents. The son felt that his mom was always bugging him about taking his medications. They agreed to keep the medicines in the kitchen cabinet. This way the parents could monitor when new prescriptions needed to be ordered. The frequency for refills of medications used daily was an established pattern. Allergy flare-up medications were on hand when needed. Since the parents ordered the refills, they would be able to tell how their boy was doing. They further agreed that as long as the son took the required amount of medications they would not question him. Since the teen wanted the independence, they decided that he would request to see the doctor if his problems became worse.

If you have a teen acting up in some way, such as not taking medicines and becoming ill, or overmedicating for attention, there are several options. You can advise the physician what is going on and suggest that your child see the physician alone. If so, make an agreement with your teen on how you will get information, following the visit, on the treatment plan. Even if you have permission from your child to talk to the doctor, never do it without involving the youngster in the discussion. This is important for two reasons: you do not want to take responsibility that is not yours, and you do not want to betray the confidentiality that exists between physician and patient. It is important that you convey your support and that you are there when needed. If your teen does not want you to talk with the doctor, make an agreement that has limitations, deciding on the limit at which you believe you need to be involved. For example, the two of you might agree that as long as your teen takes medicines as prescribed and keeps up with school and social activities, you will remain off the team. It should be clearly understood that there will be a meeting with the doctor if the limits are not met.

Another option may be to encourage your teen to participate in a teen support group. There are a number of different types of groups to choose from. If you have a child with asthma, your local American Lung Association may be able to recommend a group. Your community healthcare services may sponsor a group for teens with respiratory problems. There are also teen therapy groups run by psychologists that would be helpful.

If you feel your teen is out of control, a one-to-one visit with a psychologist may be necessary. Again, you will need to negotiate how you and your teen will determine what the plan is for improvement. Whatever actions you and your teen decide to take, you should allow confidentiality on the issues between your youngster and the physician, psychologist, or support group. It is important to listen and support but not to pry for information.

22

DETERMINING WHAT TO DO ABOUT ALLERGENS

Avoiding allergens forces a lifestyle change and when the allergic person is a child, the family is affected. Your physician will help you determine what changes need to be made first, based upon what allergies your child has and the severity of them. You need to think about the expense and disruption to your home and family.

Using the results of the skin tests, investigate where you can find the responsible allergens in your home environment (see Key 26). Then, once you find them, set priorities on the changes you want to make. For example, if your child is going to have allergy shots that include dust mite and house dust, first pay attention to the child's bedroom, since one third of the day or more is spent here. After making the recommended changes, wait to see how well your child does. Between the shots, medicine, and bedroom changes, no more measures may be necessary.

If your child continues to have problems or if you know your home needs other changes, start slowly to make them. Again, set priorities on what you can afford and what seems to be the most important problem. Sometimes, the problem is clearly not in the home. Make a trip to school or other places where your child spends much time. If your child is

56

napping at day school on an old wool carpet, that may be the only major source for trouble.

How much meeds to be done will depend on the total allergies that your child has and the degree of their potency. For instance, if your child is allergic to tree, grass, and weed pollens as well as molds, you need worry only about molds. You can control mold in the home. The shots will help control the reaction to pollens.

If your child is allergic to the family pet, pollens, and environmentals, pay attention to eliminating the environmentals. You can restrict the pet to outside. Between the allergy shots and the changes you have made, maybe you can keep the family pet.

Your physician can guide you on setting priorities based on the results of the skin tests, but he or she is not likely to come to your home.

Some parents become overconcerned about the environment, with the result that the home begins to look like a clinic. This is rarely necessary and is the sign of an overfocus on the allergic condition. The following Keys will show you some ways to eliminate or control troublesome environmental allergens of concern.

23

WHAT IS HOUSE DUST?

House dust is a substance unique to each home. It is the breakdown of various materials and includes fabric lint, pet hair or dander, dust mites, and other insect parts. Dust from outside, which feels gritty, is not the same as house dust. Because every family has different fabrics and furnishings, each home has its own unique dust.

As animal and plant fibers break down, they form dust. These fibers may include flax, cotton, silk, wool, kapok, and many more. In order to eliminate these fibers from the home environment, you must learn to identify them. If your child has a mild to moderate allergy, eliminate these fibers from only the bedroom. However, if your child spends much time in the family room, you might want to consider eliminating dust-making fibers in that room as well. The idea of balance comes into play in determining how many changes to make.

Have you ever noticed particles in a ray of sunlight? What you see in the light is only a fraction of what is really there. The dust that causes allergies cannot be seen. The visible particles breakdown to invisible particles. There are more than seven thousand of these particles, which are invisible to the naked eye, in a space no bigger than a pinhead.

Sleeping and decorative pillows are frequent sources of dust. Pillows filled with kapok, flax, or cotton are known dust makers. If your pillows do not have content labels, by pinching the pillow and moving your fingers back and forth, you may be able to determine what the filling is. Synthetic fibers feel slick and smooth. In a down pillow, you can feel the hard parts of feathers. Sometimes you can feel the seeds in kapok or flax. Cotton is harder to figure out; however, it doesn't feel as smooth as the synthetics. Foam pillows can harbor molds, and over time, break down and produce dust as well.

Dust balls under the bed are the telltale signs of dust that causes allergies. A room conditioned to control dust will not have dust balls under the bed. Dust that you see on the furniture may or may not be house dust. Wipe your hand over it. If it is gritty, it is dust from out-of-doors. If it is gray, soft, and fluffy, it is house dust formed from the breakdown of fibers. If you have an electronic air cleaner that is not functioning properly, you might see a whitish dust on the furniture.

Once you have conditioned your home to control dust, you should keep the windows closed. Dust should not build up on furniture for seven to ten days. In homes with filter systems in addition to allergy control, you will not see this build up for about a month.

24

THE MIGHTY MITE

The house dust mite is a very important cause of allergy symptoms in the home. This little critter can be seen with a magnifier in furniture and bedding. Since dust mites thrive on skin scales and dander, any place a person or pet sits or sleeps may have them.

House dust mites live for about thirty days. As they multiply and die, their body parts become part of the dust in your home. Current thinking is that their waste or feces are the most allergenic part of house dust. Mites can go into a dormancy state if conditions are not right. This may last over a hundred years. They are abundant in humid, warm climates, but furnishings in a cool climate may also provide the right environment. A person who sits in a particular chair every day may create a warm environment where mites can thrive. Since they are so difficult to eliminate, it is very important to condition furnishings so they do not flourish. One way is to create a barrier between you and their environment. For example, by encasing a mattress, you create a barrier. Furnishings can also be treated with chemicals that eliminate mites. (See Key 31 for more information.)

25

~~~~~~

POLLENS AND MOLDS

Pollens that cause allergy symptoms are not from plants with beautiful flowers. Although you frequently hear the term *rose fever*, roses seldom cause allergy. The roses are not the problem—they just happen to be in bloom when there are allergy symptoms. Actually, a nearby tree, weed, or grass is the real culprit. These plants just happen to pollinate at the same time that roses are blooming. Showy flowering plants are usually bee or insect pollinated. Flowers that do not produce great amounts of pollen do not cause allergy symptoms.

Plant vary according to climate, altitude, and latitude, and certain areas of the world are worse than others for people with pollen allergies. For example, countries near the equator do not have an abundance of airborne pollens because the humidity makes pollen too heavy. (As a result, insects pollinate the plants.) To ensure pollination in the drier, cooler climates of North America, a plant or tree must produce millions of pollen grains. These grains are light and shaped for flight so they can travel great distances. Therefore, the exposure of an allergic person who is sensitive to a particular pollen may be many miles from the plant, weed, or tree that produced the pollen.

Allergenic pollens produced by trees, weeds, and grasses occur during specific seasons. The olive tree, for example, pollinates every May in Southern California. Grasses pollinate in the late spring in the East and year-round in the Southwest. Exact weeks that trees, grasses, and weeds pollinate have been published for all areas of the country. In every area there are slight differences in the pollen seasons depending upon the climate, altitude, and latitude. The Hollister-Stier Laboratories have published these seasons for twenty-one areas of North America, and have given permission to reprint the list in the *Allergy Environment Guidebook*, mentioned on page 169 of this book.

Because allergenic pollens are so abundant and well-shaped for flight, worrying about the plants in your own yard may be only part of the answer to allergy problems. Tree-lined streets of elms in another neighborhood are more significant because each one is producing millions of pollen grains. The air around these neighborhoods will have very high pollen counts. If your child has an elm allergy and plays near the tree that produces pollen, you can expect symptoms. But except for those few weeks that the tree is pollinating, your child should not experience allergy symptoms from elm trees.

Molds also have seasons when they are excessive in the air. These mold seasons occur around the same time each year, mostly along the East Coast, the Gulf Coast and the Great Lakes. Again, depending upon the area, the seasons are different.

Molds are also significant in households everywhere. If there is dampness and a mild temperature, there will be molds. We are all familiar with mold around a shower. Sometimes you can smell a musty odor but you cannot see any mold.

If your child has tested positive to molds, you might want to test your home to see if molds are a problem. Your physician will tell you how to expose mold plates to quantify the molds. After the mold plates are exposed to the home air, they are taken to a laboratory. After a few days, molds grow on the plate. Each mold is identified, and the prevalence of mold in your home is based on how long the mold plate was exposed to home air. Sometimes it is difficult to determine the existence of a significant mold in a home. This requires some detective work. Molds will grown under leaking sinks or appliances. Sometimes closets or storage areas can harbor molds. To give you an idea where molds grow, here is a partial list:

- Closed areas—attics, basements, closets, homes closed up during vacation
- Damp areas—bathrooms, laundry, carpet pad on cement slab, leaking windows or roof, vaporizer
- Foods—bread, moist leftovers, opened food
- Furniture—antiques, furniture from a flood, foam bedding
- Special conditions—homes not conditioned for good allergy control, old homes, water seepage, barns, farms, hay bales, mulch piles, agricultural crops

When you begin to find allergen sources in the environment, you do not need to be overwhelmed. If you understand what sources are most significant, you can figure out what needs to be done in steps. Since it takes some experience to identify sources for allergies, use the environmental assessment in Key 26 as a guide.

26

THE ENVIRONMENTAL ASSESSMENT

The environment for the allergic child includes the home, the school, and the out-of-doors, as well as lifestyle activities (diet, sports, church activities, hobbies, spectator activities etc.). To help you set priorities where sources of allergy are the most important, an environmental assessment can be done to give you an overview. Using the skin test sheet as your guide, you can identify sources that require change. From there you will see what you want to do first. The most important room to condition is the child's bedroom. If you have forced air heating or air conditioning, filtering the air in the home is the next most important step. From there on, how extensively you make changes will depend upon the severity of the allergy and the response of your child to the measures already taken.

Assessment Checklist

Location

Prevailing Wind. Identify sources of problems in the prevailing wind, such as traffic, industry, cultivated farmland (name the crops), a large body of water, marshlands, a grove of trees, a golf course, fields, or open space. Identify the pollen seasons for the trees, weeds, or crops. Find the open spaces that lie in the path of the wind to your home. Are there weeds and grasses growing there?

Home Site. Identify possible sources of allergens:

_____ Rural (List any agricultural fields, farms, etc.)

_____ City (Name trees, weeds, or plants that dominate.)

———— Adjacent fields (Name weeds that predominate.)

———— Nearby ditches (Indicate if large damp areas exist.)

———— Bulldozing or large construction projects in area (Indicate if this is a new growth area and if construction will be going on for some time.)

———— Wind exposure (Are there irritants or allergens in the wind from pollutants, agriculture, pesticides, industry, heavy traffic, etc?)

———— Canyon site or nearby canyon (Name plants or trees.)

———— Large areas of repeated plant landscaping—i.e., bermuda grass, trees that line the streets, shrubs common to most of the neighborhood, etc.

———— Nearby stables, chicken pens, or other animal-enclosures

———— Other findings:

Home

Construction and Maintenance. If construction materials in the home require frequent maintenance, investigate the products used to recondition. Are substitutes available for the products that are known to cause trouble? For example, can vinyl siding or stucco be applied to the house rather than a new coat of paint?

———— Are insecticides used around the foundation?

———— Is the foundation of cement? If yes, is the slab sealed with plastic? If not, check the cement for dampness. (Occasionally, cement foundations are damp because of leaking pipes.)

———— Is the foundation above ground? If yes, is the underside of the home sealed? Vents should be sealed to prevent openings around them.

———— Is there an attic? If yes, are there any vents, pipes, or openings that share air with the interior of the home?

Forced Air System. Many of these systems draw air from places that contain allergens.

_____ Is there forced air heating? If yes, are cold air intakes drawing air from the attic, from beneath the home, from outdoors, or from the basement?

_____ Is there forced air refrigeration?

_____ Is there an electronic air cleaner? If yes, when was it last serviced and checked for efficiency?

_____ What type of mechanical filter is used in the system? How often is it changed or cleaned?

Products Used in the Home. List all the cleaning products you are using and the ingredients. Are they scented? Are they aerosol? List all the toiletries and cosmetics used in the home. Do the labels indicate possible allergens or irritants? Are the products scented? Do you use mitocide on the carpet, chairs, or other places?

Washing Methods for Bedding and Clothing.

_____ Are blankets washed every four to six weeks?

_____ Is the bedspread washed every two months?

_____ Are sheets washed weekly?

_____ Are sheets treated with a fabric softener?

_____ What brand of soap or detergent is used?

_____ Is soft water used to wash clothes? If no, is laundry soda or a water softner like Calgon added to the wash cycle?

Allergy Sufferer's Bedroom. (If the entire home requires allergy control, all these items should be removed from each room. This may be necessary if there is a forced air or air conditioning system, or if the homemaker has allergies.)

_____ Is the fill in pillow(s) foam, feathers, or a plant fiber? If so, are the pillows encased in nonporous, zippered covers?

_____ Does the mattress have a nonporous, zippered encasing?

_____ Is the box spring encased?

_____ Are blankets a tight-weave synthetic fiber?

_____ Is the bedspread made of and filled with synthetic fiber?

_____ Are sheets a fine weave such as percale, or at least 50 percent polyester, nylon, or satin?

_____ Are there any articles on the bed such as backrests, animals, or toys? If yes, are they filled with a synthetic fiber?

Furnishings. List each piece of furniture in the bedroom and indicate if it has any of the following:

_____ Is the upholstery fabric animal or plant fiber?

_____ Is the furniture ornate or does it contain many holes or crevices to harbor dust (rattan, carved or layered wood)?

_____ Is the finish of the furniture rough and not easily damp cleaned?

_____ Is the furniture oiled? If yes, does the oil contain cottonseed oil or tung oil?

_____ Are aerosols part of the furniture conditioning or cleaning?

_____ If furniture creams are part of the conditioning program, what are the ingredients?

Other Items. List other items in the bedroom that may attract or make dust.

_____ Lamp shades (Fabric?)

_____ Wall decor (Wallpaper?)

_____ Decorator pillows (kapok, cotton, flax fill?)

Windows

_____ Broken or cracked?

_____ Air leaks? Is weatherstripping wool or another fiber?

_____ Damp or decayed wood around window?

_____ Does moisture form on the window and run down to the sill? If yes, how is sill kept dry?

_____ Are there mold stains around the window, wall, or floor?

_____ Does the window in the bedroom always remain closed?

Window Treatment

_____ Shades? Washable?

_____ Shutters? Smooth enamel finish?

_____ Drapes? Washable? Dry-cleanable? Are they washed or cleaned frequently, even if they cannot be removed?

_____ Vertical blinds? Are they damp cleaned frequently?

_____ Other type window covering? Can it be damp-cleaned?

Floor

_____ Tile? Is the grout sealed with silicone?

_____ Sheet flooring? If not vinyl or sealed with polyurethane, is the floor smooth and nonporous?

_____ Wood? Is the surface sealed?

_____ How is the floor cleaned? Are any strong chemicals used?

_____ Carpet? Are the pile and fiber suitable for good allergy control (synthetic cut pile or tight weave with synthetic backing)?

_____ Carpet pad? (Pad should be a solid synthetic material.)

Animals and Other Pets. List household pets. Indicate if these pets come into the home. If so, are they restricted to one area or room? Is this area closed off from the rest of the house? It should not share air with the rest of the home. For example, is there an open doorway or a cold-air intake from the forced air heating system in this room?

Lifestyle

_____ Does your child take natural vitamins (cod liver oil, herbs)?

_____ Does your child do any cleaning? (Cleaning should be done with a damp cloth only.)

_____ Does he or she have a hobby or activity that results in a chemical exposure? What are the chemicals?

_____ Does your child mow the lawn or is she exposed to freshly cut grass?

_____ At preschool or school, is your child around any of

the items covered by this assessment? (If you have a pre-school child, review the area where your child naps.)

_____ Are there allergens at places where your child spends time (church or temple, friend's home, etc.)?

_____ Does anyone in the household smoke?

_____ Is your child exposed to adults smoking at a friend's home or during some other activity?

Once you have completed the assessment, you have an idea on how to identify allergens. Now you will want to prioritize the most important changes. Changes may include either eliminating or conditioning the allergy sources. You can condition surfaces by sealing them—for example, by applying a polyurethane coating to paper wallpaper or encasing a wall hanging behind glass. There are also chemicals to retard the formation of dust in fabrics. These are discused in the next few Keys.

27

ELIMINATING HOUSEHOLD ALLERGENS

Whether you eliminate a household allergen or recondition it, you have embarked upon a lifestyle change. You will find that you may be using different cleaning agents, toiletries, and other chemicals. Whenever you purchase an item, you will think about its potential for creating dust in your home. Before going on vacation or to an event, you will think about any potential allergens involved for your child and make plans to ensure a good time.

As you begin these changes, there are some basics that apply to all families with allergic children. They relate to the air quality of your home. One rule is to remove all aerosols from the home. These include hair sprays, furniture cleaners, room deodorants, and insecticides. The fine particles from these aerosol sprays migrate to other parts of the home. They cannot be restricted to one area.

Some parents think that confining smoking to one room of the home will not expose their child to the smoke in another area of the home. However, these fine particles stay in the air for long periods. Smoking over time also leaves a film on surfaces in the home. Worst of all, it travels through the forced air ducts throughout the home. Recent research indicates that secondhand smoke may be worse than smoking. Insist on a "no smoking" home. The American Lung Association has a variety of signs you can put on your front door or in the home.

The introduction of new furnishings or decorative fibers can cause symptoms. There is a process called "off-gassing" that can be irritating to someone with a sensitive respiratory tract. Chemical gases are released from the fibers as they dry. This off-gassing can go on for days or weeks, depending upon the size of the item. The introduction of new fibers into the home should take place during dry, warm weather. The windows should remain open for up to two weeks.

Newly purchased fabrics will frequently contain formaldehyde. By washing the fabric, you can remove the formaldehyde. This is especially true of fabrics for sewing.

Some perfume and scented products can cause symptoms. By purchasing nonscented toiletries, you can avoid this problem. Perfumes are notorious for causing allergy symptoms. It is best to try samples before purchasing. Keep in mind that on one day a perfume may not cause trouble because your child has good control of the allergies. On another day, an exposure to both a cat and the perfume will cause symptoms. The balance concept affects everything we use.

Pesticides are present in practically every household. The chemicals in pesticides do not break down quickly; therefore, they can remain active for many years. With the lack of ultraviolet light inside a home, this process takes even longer. Insecticides can build up, making an indoor exposure dangerous. The ideal way to control household insects is to use natural products. Many insecticide services use products that you do not want to expose yourself or your child to. To control pests, there are several safe solutions. Some of the old home remedies are mentioned here.

Boric acid mixed with flour, sugar, and cornmeal can be spread along baseboards to eliminate *cockroaches*. The roaches walk through this mixture. Later they lick their legs to groom. Soon they die by drying. There are other nontoxic products that do the same thing. The contents label should state silica aerogel. Spreading bay leaves, dried cucumbers, or dried garlic under cabinets will repel cockroaches. Commercially available sticky products trap roaches in a box.

Fleas are a constant problem for pets during the warm weather. A number of options are available. Pyrethrum powder, a botanical insecticide from dried flowers, paralyzes fleas. After applying the powder, place a newspaper under your pet for the fleas to drop onto. The newspaper can then be burned. There are a number of other tips to eliminate fleas. One is to walk around the house with fuzzy white socks. After the fleas get caught in the yarn, you can drown them by soaking the socks in water. Another method is to make a mixture of boiling water and sliced lemons, let it sit overnight, and then sponge your animal with the potion, thus killing the fleas. It is also important to vacuum frequently to get rid of flea eggs and larvae. Salt in the vacuum cleaner bag will ensure that the fleas trapped in there die.

Traps are still the safest method to rid the home of *rats* and *mice*. The stronger insecticides or gases used by insecticide services can cause asthmatic and allergic symptoms.

Fumigation with toxic chemicals does not affect underground *termite* nests. To avoid these chemicals, contact a service that uses liquid nitrogen, electricity, or hot air. The service will also give you ways to detect and avoid termites in the future.

To avoid using poisons to eliminate or repel *mosquitoes*, some people claim oil of citronella helps. However, it can cause symptoms in sensitive children. A bug light outside the door will help stop mosquitoes from coming into the home. Eating garlic or rubbing apple cider vinegar or crushed parsley on the skin will also repel them.

Everyone fights *ants* and has probably learned to keep foods that attract these insects in the refrigerator. When ants are active, you can spread coffee grounds or cucumber peels behind cabinets. If this does not repel them, you can crush handfuls of mint where they enter the home. If you rub the door sill or tile counters with camphor or oil of cloves, ants will not come into the kitchen.

Recently nontoxic insecticides have been introduced in the market. Beware of the nontoxic label because each state regulates labeling in a different manner. Pyrethrum and soap mixtures are good substitutes for insecticides for house plants and in the garden. Pyrethrum, however, can cause allergy in some people.

28

CLEANING TIPS

There are several cleaning agents available that are natural products. There is normally no need to buy the potent cleaners that put irritants into the air. Also, many of the old home remedies are inexpensive and can do a good job.

To control molds and bacteria, there are disinfectants that are very useful and that do not leave fumes in your home. Disinfectants that are colorless and odorless compounds that are effective at all temperatures are the best to use. Select products that have benzalkonium chloride or n-alkyl benzyl ammonium chloride on the label. Your pharmacist can help you.

Liquid chlorine disinfectants are relatively inexpensive, readily available, and effective at all temperatures. The label should state that the product contains 5.25 percent sodium hypochlorite. Bleaches should be limited to small areas with good ventilation. The strong-scented pine oil or phenolic disinfectants are effective, but the strong scent can cause symptoms and there is no need to use them with odorless compounds available.

Cleaning cycles are important to controlling allergens. Start with the following cleaning routines. You may find that you will need to shorten or lengthen the times depending upon your child's symptoms. Walls should be damp-wiped every four to six months, more often if there are symptoms. Blankets and bedspreads should be washed every four to six weeks. Floors should be damp-mopped or vacuumed twice a week. Furniture, shelves, or woodwork should be damp-wiped weekly. By staggering the cleaning tasks, you can do a little bit on a continuous basis. Once you have your routines, you may find that you actually have less housework because nothing ever gets very dirty.

Over time, soaps, fabric softeners, starch, and fabric conditioners build up in your laundry, making clothes look dull and gray. These substances can be removed with the proper use of sodium combinations such as Calgon or baking soda. If you have soft water or water-conditioning equipment, washing clothing once a month with one cup of Calgon or baking soda will keep your laundry residue-free. If you do not have water-softening equipment or naturally soft water, water-softening chemicals should be added during the rinse cycle.

If you have soft water, use biodegradable soap or detergent in very limited amounts; follow the directions. With hard water, a low suds detergent is usually the best choice. Avoid detergents with additives or conditioners unless they are softeners such as baking soda. Sometimes, the conditioners coat the fabric to leave it soft but a residue remains. Do not use liquid fabric softeners in your wash. The fabric softener sheets can also be a problem due to the scent. Your laundry will be soft if the rinse cycle removes the residue.

If your child helps with chores, it is best to avoid using dry cloths when cleaning storage areas, sweeping, or dusting. Instead use silicon-treated mops or cloths, or damp or wet cloths.

There are chemical dust retardants on the market. One brand is Allergex. These products can be used in areas where you cannot afford to replace a natural fiber item with a synthetic one.

For shiny floors, use acrylic liquids that are quicker and safer than paste wax products. Paste waxes discharge furmes for several days and produce fumes that can trigger allergic reactions.

Use full-strength liquid fabric softener on surfaces that collect dust, such as heater grills. Venetian blinds, lamp bases, or decorative grills or screens can be coated with the softener, which creates a smooth, slick surface that repels dust. If you have wall surfaces that catch dust, wipe a diluted softener solution on the walls.

Use adhesive vinyl-coated paper to line rough-textured drawers or closets. You can wipe them when you do an annual cleaning.

By now you see the point: cleaning can be done using the old standby products and still be relatively easy. There is normally no need for the fancy cleaners that put chemicals into the environment and can trigger symptoms.

29

HOT SPOTS

Any place in the home that is unused or that is used only as a storage area is a potent source for old dust. Old dust is the most antigenic dust, especially when there is a lot of it. An attic, for example, often contains dust that has accumulated undisturbed for years.

Even if your attic space is unused, check that there are no openings from the attic into the home. It is not unusual for vents to exchange air with the home. For example, there may be an opening in a hallway so that hot air can move upward into the attic and out of the interior of the home. Or air intakes in forced-air heating systems may draw air from attics. Building codes may require fresh air to be pulled into the system, and the contractor has used the attic for that purpose. If these ducts go through the attic, check the workmanship. Sometimes seams open up or ducting is too loosely fitted.

Basements can create several problems. Since they tend to be areas not used often by the family, old dust exists there. The primary problem, however, is mold caused by dampness. It is important that walls do not directly touch the soil unless there is watersealer or plastic sheeting material on the outside. Sealing the inside walls is just as important. Watersealing paint or a nonporous surface like vinyl wallboard or vinyl cloth will stop moisture.

The basement floor should have the same treatment to assure that no moisture is coming from the soil. There is an interesting example where two children in the family were having constant asthma. The parents had followed all the directions for medications and good allergy home control, but nothing worked. The physician ordered an environment study. The home, built on a hillside, had the back wall of the lower floor against the soil. The other three sides consisted of walls and windows. A musty odor throughout the home indicated molds were extensive. A large Japanese pool ran along the front of the home. The wall against the soil has been sealed against moisture and presented no problem. It was important to see if there was moisture coming from the slab floor. After the carpet was pulled up, fine lines in the floor revealed dampness. Water from the pool had traveled through the pool cement that continued as part of the slab floor. The family watersealed the floors and then put down vinyl flooring. The moisture barrier created by installing the vinyl flooring solved the problem.

Potted plants in the home need not present mold problems. There are products you can put in the soil to inhibit the growth of molds. However, dry-flower arrangements can cause problems because they become dust producers. Also, if weeds and grasses compose the bouquets, there may be problems, especially if they are not completely dry. Many decorative flowers and leaves have strong scents, such as eucalyptus, that will cause symptoms.

The attractive scented potpourri balls made of dried petals, herbs, and spices also can cause problems. The scent can permeate the whole home. As the potpourri deteriorates over time, dried particles are wisped into the air whenever someone passes.

Fresh cut flowers are not a problem unless the water becomes stagnant. A half teaspoon of bleach in the water will prevent stagnation. Some flowers that are related to botanical families of weeds may cause symptoms. For example, chrysanthemums belong to a family that has both weeds and flowering plants that cause allergy.

Garages can contain many allergens. It is best that your child not play in this area unless you have taken allergy control measures. Some children, however, have hobbies that require time in the garage. In this case, it is best to build cabinets for all storage items, or purchase plastic storage boxes instead of cardboard. If the garage is painted with enamel or the room is finished with wallboard or paneling, it can be a suitable place to spend time.

Bathrooms and laundry areas may have moisture problems. It is important that water drains quickly and that no puddles form, because dampness attracts molds. To control moisture, clean the tile surfaces and grout thoroughly. Allow to dry and then apply a silicon sealer. Cement surfaces can be sealed with a special sealer for cement. If water cannot be absorbed and is not allowed to stand, you will be able to control a significant source of moisture. Use a heater and an exhaust fan whenever hot water is used. The area should then remain dry.

Other hot spots are discussed in Keys that relate to the lifestyle of your child, such as play, camping, vacations, and holidays.

30

HOME AIR QUALITY

To control the quality of the air in the home, the windows must be closed and allergens and air pollutants must be treated or eliminated. It is important to understand that air pollutants actually build up in the closed home and that air within a closed home can be more dangerous than the air of a large city during an air-pollution alert. There are several measures, however, that can be taken to help to ensure clean air in the home.

Three methods can help control air pollutants. First, the source of pollution can be controlled by removal, substitution, or treatment. A gas water heater, for example, is vented so the combusted gases are removed from the home. Sometimes decorating materials that do not give off gases while drying can be substituted for substances that pollute the air. For instance, use of glass bricks instead of reconstituted glued wood eliminates that particular air pollutant source. This book offers several examples on how to treat fibers so they will not create or harbor dust.

Second, ventilation can very effectively reduce air pollutants in the home. Usually air from outside the home can blow inside and reduce gases or allergens. However, if allergens need to be controlled, open doors or windows may not be desirable. In these situations, forced-air heating, air-conditioning systems, or fans can move air.

The third and best way to control the quality of the air in a closed home is by filtering or exhausting air to prevent the buildup of air pollutants. Bathrooms and kitchens have built-in exhaust fans to exhaust pollutants and moisture, but the remainder of the home will also require filtering. Of course, if you have thoroughly removed all the known allergens and air pollutants from the home, filtering may not be necessary. If you have a forced-air heating or air-conditioning system, the entire home's air is mixed, and if you cannot condition the entire home, you will need to close off your child's bedroom from the forced-air system. In this case, you will want to install perimeter heat and a portable or console filter for the room.

Some basic rules can help determine how you want to filter your home and several factors will govern the effectiveness of the filter system. A filter purchased at the hardware store is not adequate for controlling allergens or air pollutants—it catches some of the large particles in the air but does not stop the smaller particles and gases. You need to consider filters that will control allergens. The chart on pages 82–83 shows what kind of filters are required for filtering specific allergens. The larger particles, such as pollen and molds, can be filtered by an efficient mechanical filter that is slipped into the forced-air system. If house dust or gases are a concern, you need to consider an electronic air cleaner or a high-efficiency particulate air filter (known as a HEPA filter) with a charcoal filter. Only these filters will remove the small dust particles that cause dust allergy.

If you want to get an electronic air cleaner or HEPA filter, it is strongly recommended that you consult an air-conditioning engineer to help design the system. If the correct modifications are not determined, drafts, inefficient filtering, and inappropriate air exchanges can result. Another important point to remember about these filters is that they do not clean your house. You must still eliminate the allergen and air-pollutant sources, and keep them out. Also, be sure to

PARTICLE SIZE

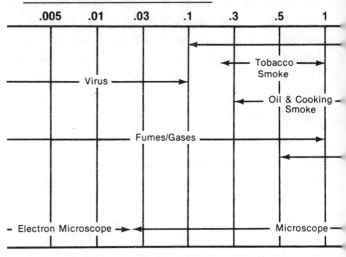

FILTER CAPABILITIES

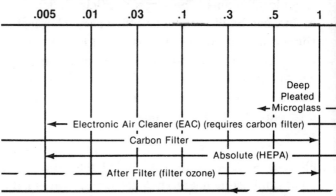

These are approximate ranges only! Efficiency is dependent upon
1) Airflow (speed) 2) Resistance in the airflow 3) Type of test used to
measure efficiency (Dust spot, State test, ASHRAE etc.)

1 Micron = 12/25,000 inch.

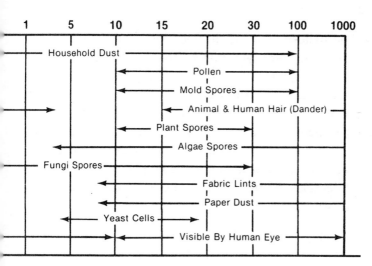

1	5	10	15	20	30	100	1000

- Household Dust ————————————→
- ←———————— Pollen ————————————→
- ←——————— Mold Spores ———————→
- ←——— Animal & Human Hair (Dander) ———
- ←——— Plant Spores ————→
- ←————————— Algae Spores ————————
- Fungi Spores ———————————————→
- ←————————— Fabric Lints ——————
- ←————————— Paper Dust ——————
- ←—— Yeast Cells ————→
- ←———————— Visible By Human Eye ————→

(IN MICRONS)

1	5	10	15	20	30	100	1000

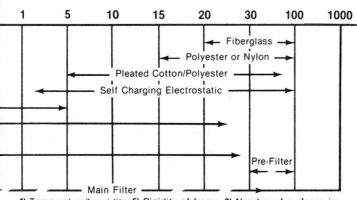

- ←— Fiberglass —→
- ←—— Polyester or Nylon ——→
- ←————— Pleated Cotton/Polyester ————————→
- ←————— Self Charging Electrostatic ————————→
- Pre-Filter ←—→
- ———— Main Filter ————

4) Temperature/humidity 5) Rigidity of frame 6) Number of surfaces in the filter 7) Cleanliness of filter (EAC inefficient if dirty, HEPA more efficient if dirty) The ideal filter has three stages (filters).

For comparison, this period (·) is 200 microns in size.

carefully follow maintenance instructions. Finally, the fan must operate 24 hours a day to be effective. If the noise of the fan is too annoying, you may not want to purchase a central filter unit.

If you believe that you do not need such high filter capability for your home, you might consider one of the filters on the chart. Polyester filter media are disposable and inexpensive and can be cut to fit the air register in your child's bedroom. You can have a frame made to fit your forced-air system and merely insert a new filter every month. The many variations of these simple filters include polyurethane foam, nylon electrostatic filter media, Dacron, pleated cotton, and pleated fiberglass. Some of these filters are disposable and others are washable.

Whether you purchase a simple filter or an electronic air cleaner or HEPA, you should plan on three components. The dirty air will first go through a pre-filter, such as one of the disposable or washable filters that can be purchased at a hardware store. This filter eliminates large particles and protects the next filter, which is one of the simple filters recommended on the chart: an electronic air cleaner or HEPA filter. After the air is clean, the last filter, the charcoal filter, filters gases out of the air.

When additional filtering capability is installed in a forced-air system, the existing blower may not be adequate for the new system. Consult an air-conditioning engineer to determine what your particular system requires.

If you do not have a forced-air system but you do want additional filtering of the air, consider one of the portable or console electronic air cleaners or HEPA filters. The size of the unit depends on the cubic feet of air in the room or your home. For a child's room, a portable unit is usually sufficient.

It is important to check your forced air system for breaks in the ducting or in the air intakes that draw air from the attic or the underside of the home. This can be a major cause of allergy symptoms. An environmental study was done in a home that had such a system, and when the ducting was examined, it was discovered that rats had chewed through the fiberglass pleated ducts (a type of ducting that is not recommended). Nests were found along the ducts as well as rat droppings, all of which turned out to be a very potent source of mold, mites, and rat dander. Installation of new ducts was required; an exterminator was called in to eliminate the rats and the underside of the home had to be cleaned.

The names of some companies that sell filters, filter media, and baseboard perimeter heat are given on pages 163–167. These products serve as examples for what you might want to consider. The expensive filters may not be necessary, however, if you live in a climate that does not require forced air heating or air conditioning, and if you have followed good allergy environment control measures.

31

~~~

YOUR CHILD'S
BEDROOM

The bedroom is the most important room in the home for allergic children. Since a child spends one third of his or her day sleeping, it is essential to condition the bedroom for good allergy control. There are three basic rules:

1. Eliminate or contain animal and plant fibers to remove dust-making sources.
2. Have non-porous surfaces on walls and floor.
3. Control the air coming into the room.

Enclose the mattress and box spring in nonporous zippered encasings such as vinyl or rubber-type fabrics that have a solid finish. Some encasings have a fabric laminated onto the plastic to make them more comfortable. Use these encasings on all mattresses, box springs, and pillows in the room. There is a list of firms at the end of this book that sell these products (see pages 163–167).

Bedding also should be made of washable synthetics. If your child has a comforter, make certain it has a Dacron fill and not feathers, cotton, or other animal or plant fiber. The beautiful cotton quilt that Grandmother made may be filled with an allergenic product. You have two choices if you have this situation. One is to encase the quilt under glass and display it on the wall; the other is to replace the fill with Dacron. If the quilt is 100 percent cotton and not filled, wash it frequently.

Sheets can be a mixture of cotton and synthetic fabric. If the synthetic content is high, there will be less lint from the sheets. If the cotton content is high, launder weekly. Nylon satin sheets are ideal; however, the child may slide out of bed!

Bear in mind that you want to keep all the surfaces in the room nonporous. The furniture in the room should have a surface that can be damp-wiped. Acrylic enamel finishes on furniture are ideal. Plastic laminates and polyurethane finishes are also desirable.

You do not want to use cleaning sprays in this room, only damp or static dust cloths. The more plant and animal fibers you have, the more particles you will have to clean. You want to avoid spreading dust into the air. By eliminating dust making, you reduce cleaning chores.

A vinyl floor or hardwood floor finished with polyurethane is ideal. However, most homes have carpeting. This is all right if the fibers are synthetic, with a very short pile and synthetic backing. The burlap-type backings break down quickly, especially if there are water spills. The carpet pad should be a solid-type rubber, not the glued or heat-pressed particle foam. These pads break down to harbor dirt. It is very important to seal a cement slab if the rug is installed over it. Cement acts like a sponge when dampness is present. This dampness will result in molds.

Decorative vinyl or vinyl-coated wallpaper, most paints, and other hard-surfaced materials are suitable for the walls. Paper-type coverings can harbor and make dust. In addition, some of the pastes can actually support mold. The same principles apply to the ceiling. If your ceilings are acoustical, make certain they are not made of asbestos. An acoustical ceiling more than twenty years old may be made of asbestos. If you find that you have asbestos, you can spray it with a vinyl paint or sealer. The safest choice, however, is to contact a specialist to remove it.

Once the walls, floor, and ceiling have smooth, wipable surfaces, follow the same treatment for the windows. Avoid drapes or curtains that must be dry cleaned. Substitute choices include enameled shutters, vertical blinds, or vinyl shades. Washable curtains are suitable if you launder them at least once a month.

Once you have the bedroom conditioned for good allergy control, the only remaining critical factors are the air sources coming into the room. The window should remain closed. It may be necessary to install a window air conditioner for the hot weather. If you have a central forced air heating/cooling system, there are several options for controlling air coming into the bedroom. It is best to keep the door closed unless you have conditioned the entire home for allergy control. Shut the forced air vent and use an auxiliary heater or air conditioner. Cut a piece of Dacron filter media to fit the vent where air enters the room. Change the filter every month. How many of these changes you make will depend upon your child's condition.

The following suggestions apply to a child with house dust or dust mite allergy. If the allergy condition of your child is mild, only the bedroom requires changes. If the child's condition is mild and includes pollen allergies, the physician may feel that only medicine can offer comfort until the shots begin to work.

If your child has moderate to severe allergy, condition the bedroom first. Over time, rid the entire home of major sources of allergy symptoms. Review your child's activities away from home, where there may be allergy sources that are more important to eliminate than those in your home. Your doctor will also recommend medications, shots, or other measures.

A child with long-standing allergies that are influencing school work and play and who needs 24-hour coverage of medicine should of course have a bedroom with good allergy control. In addition, control measures should be taken for the living areas of the home. If the child has only pollen allergies, however, these measures are not necessary, but you will need to control the air coming into the home.

Once you have your child's room conditioned for good allergy control, you will find cleaning to be easier. For example, you will need only to damp-dust surfaces. Murphy's Oil Soap for wood is also suitable. Use no sprays, cleaners, or scented products.

The bathroom your child uses can also be a source of irritating allergy symptoms. Use odorless soap, cleansers, and disinfectants. Control moisture in the room so that molds cannot grow as quickly. Sometimes it is helpful to leave on the heater or heat lamp for a while to dry out the room.

32

REDECORATING OR REMODELING THE HOME

If you have an allergic child and are planning to redecorate a room in your home or to remodel, some problems may lie ahead.

First, when you remove old carpet or wall covering, your child should not be at home. Before the child does come home, you should clear the room by using a fan to draw air out of the window.

Once a project is underway, there are several activities and products that can cause trouble. Sanding, painting, and using chemicals should be done when your child is away from the house. Try to isolate the work area from the rest of the home. Close doors and seal air vents. Since paint and chemicals may have "off-gassing" effects for a week or more, the room should remain closed until there are no fumes.

Antiques are often major sources of allergy symptoms. This does not mean you need to get rid of them, but you should condition them for good allergy control.

If the furniture is very old, has been water soaked or has been in storage for a long period, take special care to protect against these sources of allergy symptoms.

1. Seal all surfaces (inside, underneath, and back) with polyurethane.

2. Apply a finish to the outer surfaces that is smooth and resistant to damp cleaning. Ask a furniture finisher what you can use. Be careful with oil finishes; tung or cottonseed oil may cause allergy symptoms. Use a clear matte finish of polyurethane to seal the surface.

Antique fabric is a problem because you may not want to clean it. Try to figure a way to condition the fabric so it is not a source of allergy symptoms. For example, can you display the fabric under glass as art on a wall? After cleaning a fabric, a dust retardant can be applied.

Ethnic art is often a source of allergy symptoms because of the use of natural fibers or earthen dyes. Ideally, display these items under glass. If they are of a shape or size that cannot be displayed on a wall, treat the surface. Maybe you can apply a coat of polyurethane. Chinese lacquer finishes present no problem; once the lacquer dries, it provides a good surface.

If you are building or remodeling, check to see if you can install a central vacuum system. These units do not exhaust small and old dust particles into the air. They are an ideal way to control this highly antigenic dust because they do not exhaust dust inside the home. The motor unit is usually installed in a garage.

33

PLAY—WHAT IS GOOD AND WHAT IS NOT

I f a particular activity triggers allergies, try to determine the cause. The location, pollens, molds, or the activity itself may cause symptoms.

Water activities do not usually induce allergic reactions. There is usually higher humidity around large bodies of water. As a result, pollens and air pollutants tend to settle out. If allergy symptoms begin, check to see what may be in the air. Are marshlands or large areas of grass nearby? Most water sports are good choices. However, for pollen-sensitive children, sometimes the chlorine in swimming pools can irritate sensitive airways and eyes. Occasionally, a pool may have algae growth that can cause allergy.

With an allergic child, carefully plan flying a kite and other outdoor activities. The presence of pollens you are trying to avoid will help determine what plans you need to make. If particular grass, tree, or weed pollens are active, you may want to depend upon medications to avert a reaction, or you may decide to postpone the activity for a few weeks. For example, you would not want to plan a picnic in a park with oak trees during pollen season if your child is sensitive to oak. If your child likes to play outdoor sports in an open field, discuss this with your doctor. He or she may feel that avoidance is in order until allergy shots have had time to work. On the other hand, using one of the preventive medications may keep your child from sitting on the sidelines. It is always more desirable to keep your child playing than to have restrictions.

Sometimes, restrictions make common sense. The child with grass allergy should not mow the lawn. Household chores such as vacuuming, dusting, or cleaning closets expose your child unnecessarily. There are many other chores that will not involve an exposure to allergens.

Winter sports are usually very well suited for an allergic child because there are no pollens in the air. Encourage your child to participate in cold-weather activities. If cold triggers asthma, your doctor can prescribe medication to prevent symptoms.

There are some inside activities that cause symptoms— for example, gluing model airplanes may aggravate sensitive airways and cause symptoms. Your child may not be allergic to the glue; however, any strong fume can irritate the airways.

Sometimes a child's daily ritual can cause problems. Such an example was an asthmatic child who was having attacks every afternoon. A careful review showed the condition of the child's bedroom to be ideal, and there were no obvious causes for allergy in the rest of the home. When asked about the boy's activities, the mother mentioned that he jumped on the living room sofa everyday after his nap. The environmentalist's notes indicated that the sofa fill was flax. According to the skin test sheet, the boy had a flax allergy. When the sofa was removed, the child was able to reduce his medications and get his asthma under control. The parents could have had the sofa refilled with Dacron but they chose to remove it. The sofa might not have been a problem since the boy did not sleep on it. But, with his jumping, its flax fill posed a major source of allergy symptoms.

Some children like to use cardboard boxes to build imaginary places in which to play. If the boxes are new, the child will probably not get symptoms; however, any boxes that have been used for storage will be breaking down to form dust. It is best to remove boxes over a month old from the home. This is also true of old newspapers and books.

Occasionally, children will be physically active to the extent that their giggling or laughing gets them overstimulated. In some allergic children, such excitement will trigger symptoms. You can intervene by merely changing their interest to a quieter game. You don't want to restrict, but merely balance activities.

By considering in advance the activity that your child will be engaged in, you can prepare for the activity level and exposure to cold or to an environment that may have excessive allergens. In the context of balance, you will learn when you should premedicate and when it is not necessary.

34

SCHOOL—LOOKING FOR TROUBLE

I f you find your child is having symptoms at school each day, you may need to retrace his or her steps. Review for possible exposures on the way to school, in the lunchroom, the classroom or at recess in the schoolyard. Sometimes the walk to or from school is causing the symptoms, and not the classroom.

Because you cannot expect the teacher to identify allergy sources, a visit to the classroom may provide you with clues. Some key items to look for are pets, play areas, a storage area with old papers, chemicals, or the use of perfume by a teacher or aide.

If you find something significant in the classroom—for instance, caged guinea pigs—it is unrealistic to expect the teacher to remove the pets. However, be sure to explain your child's problem to the teacher and if the pet is causing obvious symptoms, whether moderate or severe, most teachers are willing to move the cage. Your child is probably not alone with this problem. If the problem is mild, talk to the nurse about when to medicate. As your child grows older, he or she will know when to go to the nurse and what to take.

Because some children like the special attention involved in getting out of class and going to the nurse, you should discuss with the nurse the child's medication regimen. Try to arrange for medications to be taken at the beginning of break periods. If you, your child, and the nurse all know when and for what reason medications are needed, there should not be a problem. You may want the nurse to check with you when your doctor has changed a prescription.

Sometimes a physical education teacher may suspect that your child is using allergy symptoms to get out of exercise. Since some exercises aggravate allergy conditions, your physician may provide a prescription for use before exercise. Some children with moderate to severe asthma may need to be excused from physical education either part or all of the time. Discuss this with your physician. Be sure to talk with the physical education teacher about your child's condition. Most teachers can substitute another activity for your youngster during this class period. If the teacher suggests study hall, evaluate if this is best for your child. A reduced activity that discontinues social interaction with classmates may not be the best solution.

Unfortunately, at some point your child may have a teacher who assumes that the condition is all in the child's head. Some parent support groups for asthma have action plans that help parents with this dilemma. If none are available to you, offer the teacher literature on the allergic response and asthma that explains about the immune reaction. If you find there is still difficulty, you need to meet with the principal. It is up to you to give your child the loving support he or she needs to handle the situation.

35

PETS ARE STILL GOOD FOR KIDS

E very child enjoys pets and learns a lot by having one. If your child has tested positive to the family pet, there are several options to explore before giving up the pet.

The first step is to try eliminating other allergens in the home. Next, if your child has a dust allergy, sometimes allergists will add cat or dog dander to the serum used for the allergy shot. With the combination of injections, elimination of other environmentals, and medication, the pet may no longer pose a problem to the youngster.

However, if your physician tells you that the allergy is significant and the pet or pets must go, there are still some options left. Ideal pets for children with allergy include reptiles, fish, or any other pets that do not produce dander. Although these pets are not cuddly pets, children can still learn from them. They can learn about their care and about assuming responsibility.

If you do not want to part with a cat, bird, or dog, however, try the following suggestions.

Your child should never groom a pet or be near one being groomed. Also, a pet should never be groomed inside the home. Keeping your pet outdoors reduces the exposure. If your family has horses, a couple of suggestions may make it safe for your child to enjoy them. For example, horseback riding may be all right as long as your child stays away from the stable and does not help groom the animal.

Cat hair and dander can be very potent. A child with a cat allergy should not be allowed to hold the cat. Recent research indicates that bathing a cat once a week in clear water reduces to some extent the incidence of cat saliva and dander on the fur. Whether or not this works, a child with significant allergy should avoid the animal. There are also some products on the market to apply to your pet that control the exposure. Your physician can give you further information.

Some caged pets such as birds, hamsters, or mice must remain inside the home. In these instances, the cage should be in a room that does not exchange air with the rest of the home. A back porch, basement room, or special area is a good choice if it can be isolated from the rest of the air in the home.

It is hard for sisters and brothers to give up a pet because their sibling has an allergy. A partial solution, if the allergy is moderate to severe, is to remove the animal(s) from inside the home.

36

SMOKING AND AUDIENCE ACTIVITIES

Smoking not only aggravates allergy conditions, but can provoke reaction in nonsmokers who are allergic to tobacco or the smoke. It is best for everyone's health not to permit smoking in the home. Smoke stays in the air even when you cannot see it. It moves from room to room and leaves a film on furniture, walls, and floors.

If your child is sensitive to smoke, check the activities in which she participates. If adults are allowed to smoke in the area, you can request there be no smoking. If you have a caregiver who smokes, change to someone who has a smoke-free home. Sometimes your child's friend's parents smoke. If they do, encourage your child to bring the friend to your home, or suggest they play outside.

It is not unusual for an allergic child to develop symptoms while involved in audience activities. Cigarette smoking in audiences can be detrimental to allergic children. Dust kicked up from wood floors in the school gym or audience hall can also induce symptoms. Sometimes, it is not the dust but the cleaners or wax coatings on the wood that bring on allergic reactions. Whatever the cause, have the child use a preventive medication, or else choose an alternative activity. People wearing strong after-shave lotion, perfume, or scented hair spray can cause allergy symptoms. Sometimes the odors of fast foods such as the popcorn sold in a movie theater can be irritating. Encourage your child to change seats if he or she is having a problem.

A teenager's friends may be smoking cigarettes or even trying marijuana. Most allergic children will avoid marijuana because it is so irritating. Some are allergic to it as well. Hopefully, they will be smart enough to avoid drug activities. You may need to reinforce this if you suspect that these activities are going to be a problem. Encourage your teen to participate in drug-free activities. You should also point out that medications are not "drugs."

Sometimes your child can get smoke exposure in places where smoking has previously occurred. This might be a car, a restroom lounge, or a particular room in the home of a friend. The smoke particles penetrate and adhere to all surfaces. You have perhaps noticed the filmy layer on the inside of the windows of a car driven by a smoker. Instruct your child to avoid these areas whenever possible.

If someone in your home smokes, contact the Lung Association for literature and information on how to end the hazardous health problem.

37

~~~~~~

CAMPING AND ASTHMA CAMPS

Most children do not have allergy conditions that warrant keeping them from camping. There may be some things that can aggravate allergies because your child will be out of the controlled environment. You can, however, plan for problems that may occur. Children treated for at least one year with allergy shots of pollen extracts usually do very well at camp.

Most camps have a nurse or someone who maintains the medicines. Good communication with this person is essential to ensure a satisfactory and enriching experience for your child. If the person is not a licensed nurse, check his or her qualifications and also find out what the camp policy is if a child has a health problem. If a physician in the area attends children with illness or injuries, contact him or her to make arrangements in case of illness. Your physician may want to send a letter with your child, advising the attending physician about the youngster's treatment program. This letter should explain your child's condition, usual medications, and allergens. The final paragraph should give your permission to treat in case of emergency.

Quite often, camps have old cabins or cottages. Since there are usually cleaning standards, however, old dust may not be a major problem. And since each camper brings his own gear, you have control over the fabrics and fill for the sleeping bag and pillow.

Some camps provide mattresses; these can be a problem. Check ahead to see if this is the case. Determine the size of the mattress and provide plastic or an encasing to cover it. Though there may be other mattresses in the cabin, it will still help if your child is not inhaling directly from an old mattress.

Cabin cleaning duty may include sweeping and cleaning. If it is possible, request that your child be given a different duty. Usually, youngsters like this will be asked to perform kitchen chores or help a counselor.

Canvas tents are a problem because they harbor molds. If the campers are given the option of sleeping outside under the stars, encourage your child to do so. This will avoid mold and dust common to canvas.

Some camping activities can be irritating to a child with allergies. By the time your child goes to camp, he or she has the experience to identify causes for symptoms. You might want to discuss possible exposures to avoid. For example, remind your child to stand away from campfire smoke.

Unless your child has specific food allergies that cause moderate to severe symptoms, let him be responsible for monitoring his food. If he has significant difficulty with food, you will need to talk to the cook about the menu. You may need to send your child substitute foods for days that the camp menu is not suitable.

Asthma camps sponsored by the American Lung Association or the Asthma and Allergy Foundation of America exist all over the country. These camps are staffed by volunteer physicians and allied health personnel familiar with the treatment of asthma.

A typical camp is usually one week at a mountain resort for asthmatic children ages nine to twelve. Activities include the usual camp experiences, such as swimming, archery, hiking, picnics, arts and crafts, skits, and day trips. A full medical staff is available 24 hours a day. The staff includes physicians specializing in asthma and allergy, registered nurses, and respiratory therapists.

Campers receive regular medications, respiratory therapy treatments, and nonallergenic diets as required. Most of these camps cost about one hundred dollars. For families unable to pay this much, the local Lung Association will frequently offer camperships.

38

VACATIONS AND TRAVEL

As you well know, with an allergic child you have to give thought to planning activities. Vacations require careful planning to ensure a pleasurable time.

When selecting where to vacation, the place to stay, the pollen seasons, and the climate are equally important. Depending on where you want to go, the potential problems can vary. There are some basic rules to help you select options for your vacation.

Winter vacations with a child who has pollen, mold, and dust allergies can be ideal as long as you don't stay in a rustic lodge. Spring, summer, and early fall vacations require special consideration of pollen seasons if pollens are a problem.

If you have a motor home or camping trailer, you have control over the sleeping environment. Most of these units are perfect for good allergy control. Follow the same recommendations for covering mattresses and pillows as you do for the ones at home. Most of the surfaces in a recreational vehicle are smooth and can be easily damp wiped. Only the articles you bring into the motor home or trailer have a potential for causing problems. You may find it necessary to install air-conditioning to ensure pollen-free air inside the unit.

If you are driving across country, you can select motels and hotels that do not allow smoking. Most hotels or motels now have certain floors or rooms dedicated to no smoking. Even though the newer hotels have synthetic materials in the rooms, it always pays to take your own pillow. The older lodges and hotels may still present problems for allergic persons. Unfortunately, old, prestigious hotels usually have the worst environment because of dust and molds.

When you are driving through cities with air pollution or through countryside with pollinating weeds or grasses, it is best to put on the air conditioner and keep the windows closed. Most car air-conditioning systems have the option of using heat with these units when necessary for chilly days. Using the air-conditioning system will dry the air, so make certain your child drinks plenty of water.

While you are planning your trip, ask your doctor for specific medicines to pack. It is worth having some contingency medicines. This can save time and a visit to an unfamiliar doctor or hospital. Most cities have urgent care centers where you can stop, should a problem develop. If you are traveling out of the country, carry a letter that lists medicines you have in your possession. A letter from the physician should explain your child's medical condition, along with the list of medications.

Car camping is like anything else. If the sleeping environment has good allergy control and you do not pick a place with active pollens, you should have a pretty good time. The tent, sleeping bags, or cots should all be synthetic. Avoid old canvas tents that are notorious for molds and old dust. It would be better to sleep outside one of these tents. The newer nylon or synthetic fabrics are not a problem.

Overnight train trips are all right in newer trains. Years ago the interior of a train was a miserable place for allergy sufferers, but the newer fabrics have eliminated that problem. Check to see if there are no-smoking cars.

Traveling in a foreign country is a different story. The only thing you can do to control the sleeping environment is to check ahead about the accommodations. In most countries, American chain hotels are better suited for good allergy control.

The change in schedule, the excitement of taking a trip, and different food can upset the balance for good allergy control. If this is the case, try to maintain a regular schedule for sleeping and eating. It is important that your child gets plenty of rest. If you are traveling, make certain the youngster drinks plenty of water. Airplanes and other air-conditioned places are dry environments.

39

HOLIDAYS AND SPECIAL DAYS

Holidays are notorious for causing problems. Just like the times you are on vacation, the schedule at holiday times becomes irregular. Different foods are eaten and there is excitement. Food particularly seems to cause trouble. The balanced diet is thrown off because of a higher intake of sweets. Also, during holidays there are more exposures to colorings and preservatives. Colorings may be allergens or irritants.

In a home with an allergic child, a live Christmas tree is better than a cut one. As the cut tree dries, pollen is released. It is best to have a tree in the house for only a short time. Your allergic child can help you decorate the tree, but exposure to dust and pollen can occur while removing the decorations.

Flocked or false-snow Christmas trees are a problem. There are several allergens in the contents of flocking materials. Avoid these trees.

At Easter, a child allergic to eggs can still dye them and hunt for them. For eating, you can substitute some other special food, such as a candy egg. From the point of view of pollen- and mold-sensitive children, November and December are usually good months in which to enjoy the special events of the Thanksgiving and holiday seasons.

In the colder areas, the first frost of the fall season marks the end of molds and pollen exposures. Even in the warmer climates, there are generally three to four months during which pollens are not active, usually November through February.

Good-weather holidays can coincide with pollen seasons and bee-sting exposures. Plan picnics and outdoor activities where an overexposure to pollens will not cause trouble. Take stinging insect precautions as described in Key 41.

Birthday parties can be an unhappy event if you have not planned ahead for possible problems. For example, the child's balance (see Keys 14–17) may be thrown off because of excitement. Add an allergy exposure to that excitement, and you have a sick child. Parents are often puzzled because they have not detected a food allergy, but the excitement was actually sufficient to cause a stomachache or other symptoms.

Special events at school, however, should be encouraged (depending upon the activity), but precautions may be necessary. An Easter egg hunt, for example, may result in over-eating chocolate or exposure to a pollen. This does not mean that you should restrict your child's participation—merely premedicate or save the chocolate for eating over a longer period of time.

The smoke from fireworks on the Fourth of July can irritate the respiratory system. Before enjoying that kind of show, check the direction of the wind and be sure it is not blowing from the scene of activity toward your child.

40

~~~~~~

RECOGNIZING THE CHILD WITH ASTHMA

Sometimes asthma is silent and you may be unaware that your child has a constricted airway. Since it takes about 50 percent of the airway to be constricted to hear wheezing, your child could still have asthma without wheezing.

One of the telltale signs of early or mild asthma in children is a night cough. They may have a dry cough in their sleep. Some will become tired easily. Your child may complain of a tight chest, stomachache, headache, or dry mouth. These symptoms may be part of obstructed breathing.

When a child has an asthma attack, it can be frightening for both parent and child. To give you an idea of the anxiety these children experience, breathe through a straw for a few minutes. You will soon find out how their inability to breathe properly feels. If your child gets panicky, it provokes even more anxiety. If asthma attacks are new to you and your child, encourage her to relax. Let her know that the condition is temporary and that she will be all right. If you have medication, administer it, then assure her that the medication will help in a little while. Read to your child or involve her in some other quiet activity until her breathing is under control.

Before going to the allergist for a workup, try to connect the triggers with the symptoms. Triggers can be allergens such as dust or a cat, irritants such as cold air and air pollution, emotional states such as laughing, or physical states such as exercise.

Allergy symptoms may include inability to sustain active play, coughing, or wheezing. Less obvious symptoms are stomachache, headache, or a runny nose. Some children get asthma from a viral infection. If so, they seem to get worse at the end of the illness. Other youngsters seem to have many colds, some of which may really be allergies.

As you learn about triggers for asthma, you will begin to notice specific emotional and physical changes in your child. His or her mood may change from aggressive to grouchy, to oversensitive, sad, or tired. If you see changes in mood, it is important to note them even though you cannot find a cause.

A child with active allergies will not look the same as usual. Key 3 describes the face of the allergic child, with its black circles under the eyes (allergic shiners) and gaping expression. If the child has not had allergies for very long, he or she may just look pale.

Breathing changes also become noticeable. If your child is occasionally short of breath, coughs, or breathes through his mouth, take note of the activities that precede such episodes.

Your child may complain about symptoms not connected with asthma, such as stomachaches or headaches. He may be unusually thirsty or have a dry mouth because of mouth breathing. Quick identification of triggers can speed up treatment.

41

INSECT ALLERGY

Stinging insects (Hymenoptera) that are of the most concern to allergic individuals include yellow jackets, wasps, and bees. There are other stinging insects, such as mosquitoes and fire ants, that also present risks. Children who have allergies are not at greater risk for reactions than the regular population. When these insects sting, swelling and itching occur at the site of the sting. The face can swell more than other parts of the body. A normal sting reaction results in symptoms only at the site of the sting.

Whenever the sting results in symptoms that are not restricted to the site of the sting, an allergic response is taking place. Symptoms may include swelling well beyond the site of the sting. A rash, itching all over the body, a tight throat, or difficulty breathing are a few of the possible symptoms to look for in an allergic child.

Antibodies form as the result of the first sting from a stinging insect. The potential for an allergy reaction is now there. The second sting may cause allergy symptoms ranging from mild to severe. Severe symptoms can be life threatening and they should receive immediate treatment (see Key 7).

If your child has difficulty breathing or is unconscious, call the paramedics immediately. If there is no problem in breathing and the child is conscious, telephone your doctor for emergency instructions. Your child may be having an anaphylactic reaction, the shock reaction described in Key 7. If your doctor has supplied you with an emergency kit, follow the instructions to give epinephrine. While you administer the shot, have someone call either the paramedics or the physician, depending on the child's condition.

If an asthmatic child suffers breathing difficulty after a bee sting, have the victim use an inhaler. This will give you time to get help. There is not much time, because anaphylactic reactions are almost immediate, occurring within ten to fifteen minutes.

A physician should be contacted about any sting that includes symptoms beyond the site of the sting—for example, a rash or unusual swelling. Sometimes, delayed symptoms (ones appearing more than a half hour after the stinging incident) may develop. Symptoms that appear one to ten days after the sting are unusual and require medical evaluation. These symptoms may include swelling, joint pains, hives, fever, or headache. Contact your physician on the day you notice the symptoms so that he or she can decide if it is necessary to see your child.

If you do not have a stinging insect kit, the physician will determine if one should be available in the future. He or she probably will refer you to an allergist, who may administer some skin tests for different stinging insects. After the patient's history is taken and the tests are given, the allergist will decide upon the treatment program. This may include allergy shots.

If your child is sensitive to stinging insects, avoidance of them is necessary. Prevention should become a lifestyle change. Here are some helpful suggestions:

1. Have your child avoid wearing bright-colored clothing when out-of-doors.

2. Buy only unscented toiletries.

3. Teach your child to stay away from bright or

fragrant flowers and to play some distance from bushes and water that attracts bees.

4. Have your child wear a medical alert tag, identifying the allergy to stinging insects.

5. Give the nurse or teacher an emergency kit with instructions on what to do. Even if children are oldenough to carry the kit themselves, the teacher should still be taught what to do. It is always easier to keep the kit in a specific place known to the teacher.

6. If your lawn has clover grass, keep it cut short or gradually change it over to a grass that will not attract bees.

7. If you have showy flowering plants in your garden that attract bees, slowly change over to less flowery plants.

8. Encourage your child always to wear shoes especially outdoors.

Some of the more common stinging insects are described in the chart on page 114. Another that can cause severe allergic reactions is the scorpion. Less severe reactions can occur from bites by mosquitoes, fleas, or flies. There are two types of reactions. One is like the reaction from the skin test—a wheal or bubblelike blister that accompanies redness and itching. A delayed reaction may persist for hours or days; symptoms may include edema and intense itching. Allergy to mite, tick, spider, and flea bites also causes intense itching. Sometimes the site becomes purple in color after a couple of days. Fleas, lice, garden bugs, caterpillars, and beetles all are potential allergens.

COMMON STINGING INSECTS

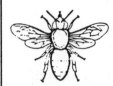

Honeybee

Honeybees Easily recognized by their small, stocky, brown, yellow, or black bodies with a round abdomen. Probably the best-known insect, honeybees are found most frequently in artificial hives, but the colonies may be found in natural nests inside the trunks of trees, under floorboards, and in other enclosed areas. The stinger differs from that of the yellow jacket, wasp, or hornet, in that it cannot be used repeatedly (the stinging apparatus is severed from the body after the sting, the stinger is left in the skin, and the bees dies).

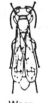

Wasp

Wasps Black or brown with yellow or white stripes and a fusiform (tapering toward each end) abdomen. The wasp can be distinguished from the yellow jacket and the hornet by its thin waist, which joins the abdomen and the thorax. Wasps are not as excitable as the other stinging insects; they usually sting only if touched or brushed while in flight around the nest. They build their nests in trees or around shelters such as the eaves of houses or porches. The nest is usually small and contains thirty to sixty insects.

Hornet

Hornets Black body with white markings on the thorax and abdomen. The face, excluding the top of the head, is also white. Hornets may be difficult to distinguish from yellow jackets, since they often have yellow markings. Hornets' nests are large, gray, or brown and are located in tree branches, under the eaves of houses, or against a wall, usually more than four feet above the ground. Hornets are considered the most aggressive of the major stinging insects, sometimes attacking without apparent provocation.

Yellow Jacket

Yellow jackets are located in the ground, often in tall grass between the walls of buildings or under stones.

Fire Ant

Fire ants Introduced from South America during the 1920s, fire ants are now well established in several Southern states. The venom of the fire ant differs from that of hymenoptera insects, in that it can produce severe local reactions or systemic anaphylactic reactions. The insect attacks by biting to secure itself, then inserts its stinging apparatus, which contains the venom. Highly sensitive patients with high levels of allergic antibodies against the venom of the fire ant are usually treated with immunotherapy.

Source: **Allergy Encyclopedia** Permission to print the above descriptions and sketches by Phil Jones has been granted by the Asthma and Allergy Foundation of America. It is from the *Allergy Encyclopedia,* out of print.

42

IMMUNIZATIONS

There has been considerable study on the risk-benefit of vaccinations. Research continues on ailments, allergic reactions, and complications that are the result of vaccinations.

Some vaccines contain antibiotics, preservatives, live cultures, or additives. At this time, the measles-mumps-rubella (MMR) vaccine is of great concern because this vaccine is grown on chick or duck embryos. Because there is a measles epidemic in several cities in the United States, all children need to be vaccinated.

Merck Sharp & Dohm, the pharmaceutical company that produces the live MMR vaccine, has the following statement in their indications for risk of reactions:

Live measles vaccine and live mumps vaccine are produced in chick embryo cell culture. Persons with a history of anaphylactic, anaphylactoid, or other immediate reactions (e.g., hives, swelling of the mouth and throat, difficulty breathing, hypotension, or shock) subsequent to egg ingestion should not be vaccinated. Evidence indicates that persons are not at increased risk if they have egg allergies that are not anaphylactic or anaphylactoid in nature. Such persons may be vaccinated in the usual manner. There is no evidence to indicate that persons with allergies to chickens or feathers are at increased risk of reaction to the vaccine.

Very few allergic children have problems from childhood immunizations. Children with eczema should not get immunizations through a school or community program until talking to their doctor. See Key 44 for information about eczema complications. Children with such sensitive skin can have skin reactions from immunizations if their skin is inflamed at the time.

Children with respiratory allergies need the annual influenza immunization. If your child is allergic to eggs, the benefits of immunization far outweigh the concern for allergic reactions. Your allergist will be up-to-date on the cultures used to produce the various immunizations.

To feel secure, get immunizations from your physician rather than from a community program. Most physicians have children at risk for allergy reactions wait in the office for fifteen minutes, the usual time for an allergic response. Sometimes physicians will advise special vaccine preparations to ensure there will be no allergic reaction.

43

^^

MEDICINE REACTIONS

Typical allergic reactions to drugs include hives, body swelling, nasal symptoms, wheezing, or skin rashes. There are also reactions that are not allergy related that include fever, or liver, kidney, or blood changes. If your child takes a medicine with known side effects, the doctor will conduct blood tests to monitor for possible drug reactions not related to allergy.

It is difficult to know when an allergic reaction will occur. Once it has, a notice will remain on your child's chart to avoid the medication. Occasionally there are no alternatives. A drug that causes an allergy reaction should be given under very controlled measures in an intensive care unit.

Drugs that often cause allergy reactions include:

Antibiotics—penicillin, cephalosporins, sulfonamides or sulfa drugs, erythromycin, and many others

Sedatives such as phenobarbital

Over-the-counter drugs such as aspirin or laxatives

Tranquilizers

Hormones such as ACTH or insulin

Anticonvulsive drugs

Iodides and bromides

Local anesthetics such as the -caines (procaine, etc.)

Vitamins also have the potential for allergic reactions, especially vitamins made from natural sources. These sources can include fish products or herbs related to weeds. Although there is no direct evidence that coloring causes allergy symptoms, it should be considered a possible source.

Most drug reactions in children appear as rashes. Sometimes it is difficult to decide if a rash is from an allergic reaction, a medication, or illness. There are so many reasons for rashes that physicians often do not find the cause. If a doctor is not available to examine the rash, take notes. Write down what your child has taken and describe the rash. Note where it covered the body. When you do see the doctor, you will need the answers to some questions. Did the rash feel bumpy? Did it itch? How long did it last? Was it red? If you have a camera, take a picture. Try to note other possible causes. What has your child eaten the past couple of days? Where was she or he playing? Has there been an illness or infection?

Antibiotics are especially suspect when a rash appears in the user. Many infectious illnesses also produce a rash as part of the illness. The physician may decide to change the medication or perhaps wait to see how the child progresses.

Some medications cause symptoms that are not allergic in nature. They may be side effects or reactions unique to the patient. Symptoms may include intestinal upset, diarrhea, headache, and many others. The doctor or pharmacist can warn you about possible side effects and what to do. You can also ask for the insert from the pharmaceutical company.

Parents of allergic children should not use over-the-counter preparations without talking first to the doctor. Experimenting wastes time and exposes the child to ingredients the doctor may want the youngster to avoid.

Aspirin needs special mention because it is a drug that parents frequently buy and administer without consulting the physician. There are several problems that aspirin can cause besides allergy. In large amounts, this drug can cause nausea, dizziness, and ringing in the ears. In aspirin-sensitive children, aspirin can cause severe asthma. Unfortunately, it is easy to give small children doses that are too large for their size. In some asthmatics, reactions may occur later. One such condition is nasal polyps, which are hard to treat. Nasal polyps are a tissue swelling or growth in the nasal passage that is related to taking aspirin. Another condition is bleeding. Someone taking aspirin will bleed more easily, because the drug causes changes in the blood. Reye's syndrome, a neurological disorder, can be caused by aspirin. There are not always warnings about some of these side effects on package inserts or labeling. Pediatricians today encourage the use of Tylenol or other anti-inflammatory preparations for fever or discomfort.

Many medications caution the user to stay out of the sun. These include acne medications such as Retin A and tetracycline, some antibiotics, some seizure medications, and medications used to control brain disorders such as psychoses and depression. If you do not apply a sun block to a child using one of these medications, a severe burn may result in a very few minutes. Since some sun blocks are irritating to sensitive skins, ask your doctor to recommend a hypoallergenic block when prescribing a medication that can cause photosensitivity.

Knowledge of immunization and medication complications resulting from the allergic condition will help you understand why it is important not to ignore allergy symptoms.

44

COMPLICATIONS OF ALLERGIES

I n describing how to recognize allergy earlier in the book, the discussion covered mannerisms that allergic children develop to relieve stuffiness and itching. There are complications that can result from any area affected by allergies.

Asthma

In the past two years, research has brought new understanding of asthma. Asthma is actually now viewed as a series of phases. The body's reactions are different in each. Asthma treatment used to focus on brochoconstriction; today inflammation is more important. Complications can be avoided by understanding what phase of asthma a child is having. Phases include a preventive phase, a warning phase, an early phase attack, and a later phase attack. Complications can be avoided by using the correct medications at the right time. A severe attack may occur if you figure your child will get better, and as a result, do nothing.

Until you learn to recognize these different phases, rely on asking your doctor about your concerns. Once an attack results in moderate to severe breathing problems, inflammation is already the major problem. The doctor prefers to catch inflammation during warning signs. Ideally, you want to try to keep your child in the prevention stage or symptom-free phase.

Don't just try a medication to see if it will work, because each phase requires particular medicines. After a day into an attack, the swollen linings of the lungs are engorged with fluid. You can put your child at risk by not giving the right drug. Remember, you can call the doctor's office for advice. Ask for the nurse; more than likely, she will be able to answer your questions. She can also quickly recognize certain symptoms that require the doctor's involvement. Don't be timid about asking questions. Once you have gone through this, you will learn to recognize warning signs yourself.

You should keep a record of the measures you are taking and the drugs you are giving your child. When you talk to the doctor, you will then be able to answer quickly and correctly. It also will help you to learn more about how your child responds to different treatment routines.

If your child has asthma and gets pneumonia, this may be the result of mucus clinging to an area in the lung that then becomes infected. You may hear the physician use the term *atelectasis*, which means there is an absence of the exchange of air in a part of the lung. Mucus tends to cling because it is often dry and sticky. If a patch of mucus clings long enough to get infected, it is called pneumonia. This complication results when mucus cannot move out of the lungs, and that is why it is so important to keep the airways clear and to control inflammation. Medications are very important in controling spasm and inflammation.

Ears, Nose, Throat, and Eyes

In Key 3, some facial characteristics of the allergic child were discussed. These characteristic signs result from constant swelling or from the effort to relieve itching or stuffiness. Deformities and chronic problems can result from long-standing allergy symptoms.

The Allergic Salute. The child who constantly pushes the nose upward in the allergic salute will develop a crease across the top of the nose.

Allergic Shiners. Allergic shiners (black circles under the eyes) result from the swelling of nose membranes from nasal allergies. Because of the pressure in the tissues, there is not proper drainage of blood vessels, thus the darkened appearance. The bags that develop contain fluid that collects under the eyes. Allergic children of any color skin will eventually have this darkened area. Even a one year old may have minishadows under the eyes. It takes about one year of nasal and sinus congestion to cause this condition.

Mouth Breathers. Because children with nasal allergies are unable to breathe through their nose, they breathe through their mouth. The gaping look is a sign that orthodontia is in their future.

Prolonged mouth breathing changes the shape of the mouth. These children will eventually get an overbite on the top as the structures become narrowed. If the overbite becomes severe, the child will require braces and oral surgery to correct the bite.

It is not clear if children with allergies rest their tongue on the roof of their mouth more than other children. The pressure of the tongue can also cause deformity. You can quickly identify a baby with this condition because you can see the tongue resting on the upper palate—it protrudes slightly. The older child may also rest his tongue on the palate but you can no longer see it.

Eye Complications. Allergic eyes are watery and itchy, and become red from rubbing. The congestion can result in thick mucus and frequent infection. If you notice a yellow to green mucus discharge, your child probably has an infection.

If your child has frequent eye problems, your physician will provide various instructions for eye care, including preventive medications.

In some allergic children, the eyes swell shut. Insect stings on the face can also cause swelling. The swelling, while uncomfortable, will not permanently impair the child's vision. Your physician will prescribe medications to prevent or reduce swelling.

Conjunctivitis, when the white of the eye or the inner surface of the eyelid becomes inflamed, can be an allergic reaction, particularly if it is recurrent. Sometimes the inner surface of the eyelid gets little bumps from long-term allergies. When studied, eosinophil cells (a type of leukocyte or white blood cell) are found in the discharge from the eye. Eosinophils are related to the allergic reaction.

Nasal Problems. Nasal allergies also can result in secondary infections from constant congestion. These children will suffer with ear, eye, and sinus infections. Sinus infections can cause infections in the lower airways.

Nosebleeds are not uncommon in children with nasal allergies. The nose swells inside, stretching blood vessels. Whenever the child irritates the nose—for example, by giving the allergic salute—the nose can bleed. Children irritated by mucus crusts frequently pick their noses. If your child is having frequent nosebleeds, talk to the doctor; there are several options to reduce or stop them. They include antihistamines/decongestants, humidification, and nasal medications that go into the nose.

Ear Problems. Some young children may have symptoms in their ears and no other signs of allergy. These symptoms frequently result from food allergy. Fluid may collect in the middle ear behind the eardrum because of swelling caused by an allergic reaction. The child then may experience pain or discomfort. The middle ear is an air space. When you swallow, yawn, or chew, air enters the middle ear. If the eustachian tube that connects it to the nasal passages swells, the air pressure cannot equalize. To keep the tube open, physicians use antibiotics or prednisone to clear the area. In addition, many physicians prescribe an antihistamine/decongestant with allergy environment instructions. If treatment does not work, small tubes inserted into the ear will drain fluid and circulate air in the middle ear. This treatment is under review to determine if longer trials of medications work as well as inserting tubes.

When you cannot avoid altitude changes, there are some considerations. Whenever you fly or when you travel in the car down a mountain, a decongestant should be given to your child at least a half hour before descending in altitude. The ears will pop when a plane climbs or when you drive up a mountain. The pain results when you descend, because the increased pressure prevents normal popping of the ears. In addition to the decongestant, it is good to give small children something to suck on. You can nurse a baby, or give an infant a bottle. A screaming child on descent is telling you there is pain. If you are driving, stop for a while to allow the ears to adjust. Small children with colds or existing ear symptoms should not fly. Older children can chew gum and do a maneuver called the valsalva maneuver. By pinching the nose closed, then gently blowing against the closed mouth and nose, the ears should pop open.

Children with fluid in their ears can eventually suffer hearing loss. This loss can occur from an ear infection or for a long period as in allergy. The hearing usually improves after treatment. It is important to keep the ears free of fluid. Sometimes fluid in the ear goes unnoticed until a hearing test at school identifies the child as having a problem. Sometimes the teacher notices a child who cannot hear or does not follow instructions. A child may act jumpy or fidgety because he or she cannot hear well. Or a child unable to hear well may be passive and inattentive.

Frequently parents do not know their child has fluid in the ear. Be alert to any complaints from your child. A child too young to talk may signal discomfort by rubbing or tugging at her ear. Older children may complain that their ears feel full or blocked. They also may make statements that their ears are popping, crackling, or making funny noises.

Tonsillectomy and Adenoidectomy. An allergic child has the same risks as the nonallergic youngster in relation to the removal of tonsils and adenoids. During the last decade, it has become the practice not to remove them unless necessary. Children get enlarged tonsils and adenoids while they are young because there are so many childhood illnesses. One of the first lines of defense, the tonsils and adenoids, grow large from overwork. After age six, these tissues begin to shrink. Only under certain conditions will a physician remove them. These conditions include:
• Frequent repeated infections of the tonsils, especially strep infection
• Abscesses in the crypts or holes of the tissue
• Recurrent hearing loss from enlarged adenoids
• Inability to swallow or breathe because of enlargement of the tissues

With all these conditions as possibilities, concerned parents tend to worry about the health of their allergic children. However, it takes time and experience to learn to recognize warning signs. Physicians and their nursing staffs answer questions all day long. When you are uncertain about anything, call. (This subject is discussed in greater detail in Key 45.)

125

Skin

If the child has some inhalant allergies such as pollens and molds, in addition to other allergy symtoms, allergy shots may be beneficial. However, in some instances, these shots may make the eczema worse.

When daily routines do not keep the skin clear, cortisone creams or a change in the skin-care routine becomes important. Sometimes steroids must be given orally for severe conditions.

These children are at risk for serious flare-ups when their skin is already reacting with redness and weeping. For example, a vaccination can cause a severe flare-up. In fact, if a family member gets a vaccination and the virus contacts the skin of the allergic child, a serious problem results. Severe inflammation can occur in this instance through bath water or bedding as well as through actual touch. Physicians will advise that no family member get a vaccination unless the allergic child's skin is clear. If a family member or caregiver has an outbreak of herpes, the same precautions are necessary. Sometimes it is difficult to find a good time to have vaccinations. In this case, the doctor may recommend that the allergic child or family member visit a relative until the risk is over.

There are other precautions that parents should observe in order to avoid flare-ups. Because perspiration causes itching, the skin should not become overheated, through either play, weather, or a hot bath. The itching starts scratching that causes the inflammation.

To control infection from fingernail scratches, fingernails must be cut each week. Daily checking of the nails each day guards against snags or dirty nails that can cause infection.

If a skin infection does occur, the child should be put on antibiotics as soon as possible.

Skin care can be frustrating, because an extensive routine is needed to keep the skin clear. There are products that help moisturize the skin during bathing. Anti-itch and moisture preparations also help to keep the skin in good condition.

Sometimes some of the recommended soaps do not work well because of hard water. Hard water will leave a ring around the tub and residue on skin and in clothes. In that case, it may be better to avoid bathing and to clean the skin with special lotions. Laundry additives such as bleach and fabric softeners can also cause problems.

Antihistamines help to decrease itch. Some of the stronger antihistamines that have sleepiness as a side effect will help to stop the scratching at night.

Because these children are so sensitive, every new soap, lotion, or cream should be tested by placing a small amount on the skin for several days. If there is no inflammation, the product is considered safe to use.

45

‸‸‸

WHEN TO CALL THE DOCTOR

U se the following chart as a guide in deciding when to call the doctor. With babies, or children who have asthma or ear problems, it is *always* wise to call the doctor. These conditions can worsen quickly and cause serious problems. Most allergy conditions are not serious, however, and it is a matter of learning enough about them so that you can feel comfortable. If you have confidence in being able to make informed decisions, you will be able to refocus on your whole family and keep a healthy balance of activity.

Problem	Up to Age 2	Age 3 and Older
Ear		
Pain	Crying and touching side of head (ear): Take to doctor or urgent care center	Complains of moderate to severe pain: Take to doctor or urgent care center
Fever	Temperature with ear pain: Take to doctor or urgent care center	Temperature with ear pain: Take to doctor or urgent care center
Hearing	Make appointment for near future if loss noted	Make appointment for near future if loss noted

Nose

Pain	Crying or fussy: Make appointment for that day	Crying, cranky, or complaining of pain: Make appointment for that day
Discharge	Yellow to green: Make appointment for sick visit for that day	Yellow to green: Make appointment for sick visit for that day
Stuffiness	Newborn babies cannot breathe without crying: Call doctor	Make appointment if it does not clear up or if it reappears
Fever	Make appointment for sick visit for that day	Make appointment for sick visit for that day

Throat

Pain	Fussy: Wait	Complains: Wait
Appearance	Red with white spots: Make appointment	Red with white spots: Make appointment
Fever	Make appointment for sick visit for that day	Make appointment for sick visit for that day
Swelling	Difficulty breathing: Take to urgent care or hospital emergency room	Difficulty breathing: Take to urgent care or hospital emergency room

Eye

Appearance	White is inflamed: Call for appointment for that day	White is inflamed: Call for appointment for that day
Discharge	1. Make appointment for future 2. Call for same day appointment if discharge is green or eyes are swollen	1. Make appointment for future 2. Call for same day appointment if discharge is green or eyes are swollen

Gastrointestinal

Colic or abdominal pain	Frequently pulls up legs and cries: Make appointment if it persists for more than day or talk to nurse	Frequently complains of abdominal pain: Make appointment if it persists for more than a day or talk to nurse
Diaherra (no illness or fever)	Call nurse for instructions on keeping your baby hydrated. Ask when to call if diarrhea continues.	If diarrhea lasts more than a couple of days, call doctor
Poor appetite	If condition lasts more than a couple of days, call doctor for instruction	If child lacks energy and looks pale, make appointment for near future

Fever and poor appetite	Call for sick visit	Call for sick visit

Chest

First time wheezing heard	Call doctor or take to urgent care	Call doctor or take to urgent care
Breathing	If tummy, area between ribs, or throat is sucked in as baby breathes: Call doctor or take to urgent care	Respirations are faster than normal: Call doctor for instructions
Fever with any of the above	Call doctor	Call doctor
Sputum	Yellow/green: Call for same-day sick visit	Yellow/green: Call for same-day sick visit

Hives

Lasts longer than 1 hour after sting; longer than 1 day, with illness	Call doctor or make same day appointment	Call doctor or make same day appointment
From food or activity	Note what child has eaten and tell doctor on next regular visit	Note what child was doing and eating

131

Sleep

Unable to sleep (unable to breathe comfortably, medicine stim- ulating child)	Call doctor or make appointment for near future	Call doctor or make appointment for near future
Symptoms of allergy at night (cough, stuffy nose)	Make appointment for near future	Make appointment for near future

Also, you should be familiar with side effects of medications. Ask your pharmacist for the warning insert for each medication. Some side effects are expected. For example, dry mouth and drowsiness are common effects of some of the antihistamines/decongestants. Nervousness and increased activity usually accompany a bronchodilator medication. If these side reactions seem to be worse than expected or if they are disrupting your child's play or sleep, call your doctor. There are different ways to handle side effects by changing dosages or medications.

46

FINDING FOOD ALLERGIES

In the early Keys, the discussion of food allergies emphasized how difficult it is to diagnose them. Skin tests can only indicate a possible food allergy. This section will provide the early steps for identifying an offending allergen.

The common food allergens are eggs, milk, peanuts, peas, pork, wheat, chocolate, corn, shellfish, and yeast. If these foods show positive on your child's skin tests, the allergist can give you avoidance information sheets that identify where you will find the offending food.

If your child's skin test results indicate that only some foods are positive, your physician probably will instruct you to avoid serving these foods. Unless your child has a history of food allergy and positive skin test reactions, and because food allergies are so difficult to determine, most physicians prefer to focus on other allergies and medication (unless a food allergy is obvious). For example, treatment may be limited to allergy shots for pollens and molds, prescriptions for medications, and recommendations for environment control. Attention to these areas quite often brings about a balance, and the foods do not throw the balance off. If you have a baby or a child with a history of food allergy, however, it makes sense to focus on a food elimination diet and identify the offending allergen.

Because so many dishes are combinations of food, it can become difficult to control the diet. There are some basic guidelines that may aid you in preparing food.

The simpler the food, the safer the choice. For example, single food dishes instead of casseroles enable you to avoid combinations of foods, one of which may contain an allergen. With homemade spaghetti sauce you can eliminate herbs found in store-bought sauces. Herbal seasonings may be botanically related to allergenic weeds. If your child has tested positive to sage, for example, you would not want to add this herb to a dish. Most children like their food plain. This may be nature's way of telling them to avoid seasonings.

Fresh frozen foods and canned foods are better than fresh foods, because processing reduces the potency of an allergen. Eating cooked fresh vegetables is better than eating raw ones.

If your child does not particularly like junk food, let him or her decide what to eat. Sometimes a food tastes funny or unpleasant because there is an undiscovered allergy involved. An example of this was a child who hated melons. But until he was old enough to talk and explain why, nobody knew that his mouth itched when he ate this fruit.

Often, preschool children are picky and do not require much food. A vegetable helping of six peas may fulfill nutritional requirements! A study conducted to see if nutritional requirements were being met had an interesting conclusion. Some young children were allowed to choose anything they wanted from the cafeteria selections. At first they gravitated toward the sweets, but after a while, they naturally began to select a balanced diet.

Trust your child's natural sense of what he or she needs. If you offer choices and a variety of foods, children usually will select what they need. If a youngster dislikes certain vegetables, it may be due to an allergic reaction he or she is not aware of.

Learn to read labels so that you become aware of what is in the food you buy. As a result, you will find you want to make your own dishes so you have control over the ingredients. Reading labels is very important when you want to avoid specific allergens. Read the labels on all prepared, packaged, frozen, canned, and dried foods. Health foods—liquids, powders, and tonics—are especially important to check because they often include ingredients that cause allergies.

Cow's milk, a common allergy food, contains more than twenty allergens. Goat's milk or canned or powdered milk will still all include these allergens. Milk elimination diets require substituting a soy product such as Mocha Mix. Some children allergic to soy milk use fruit juice on their cereal. If the label mentions casein, caseinate, whey, lactalbumin, sodium caseinate, lactose, nonfat milk solids, cream, calcium caseinate, nougat, half and half, curds, or lactoglobulin, don't buy the product.

Products with soy bean derivatives may list soy flour, soybean oil, vegetable oil, soy protein, textured vegetable protein (TVP), soy lecithin, vegetable starch, vegetable gum, or Japanese sauce on the label.

Egg may be an ingredient if you see the words albumin, egg whites, egg yolks, eggnog, mayonnaise, ovalbumin, or ova mucoid. Egg substitutes, developed to avoid the cholesterol in egg yolks, may contain egg whites or albumin.

Wheat can be present if the label states enriched flour, wheat germ, wheat bran, wheat starch, gluten, food starch, vegetable starch, vegetable gum, bran, farina, graham flour, wheat gluten, or whole wheat flour.

Corn product labels may include cornmeal, cornstarch, corn oil, corn syrup, corn sweetener, corn alcohol, vegetable oil, vegetable starch, vegetable gum, or food starch.

Labeling for beef or pork products is not good. Labels rarely include shortening, lard, or gelatin. Beef and pork products are found in combination foods, refried beans, canned foods, foods with gelatin, and frozen dinners.

There are two ways to discover an allergenic food: one is to have the child follow an elimination diet; the other is to keep the child on a diet of low-allergy foods. During either of these diets, it is very important to read labels and to be aware of some facts.

Sometimes, you may feel that just a little bit of a particular food on one day will not matter. However, adding even a very small amount of a suspect food can make the elimination diet worthless. Research data indicates that it takes the body three weeks to heal from a reaction. Since you will not know what triggered the reaction, you should really restart the diet.

Before you have the youngster begin a low-allergy or elimination diet, keep a diet diary for a few weeks. Most of the time nutritional needs can be met; however, the diet should be reviewed with your doctor. The diary should list hours of the day and have two columns, one for foods eaten and one for symptoms. For example:

	Foods/Ingredients Eaten	Symptoms
7:00 am	_____	_____
	_____	_____
	_____	_____
8:00 am	_____	_____
	_____	_____

Continue by listing the hours that your child normally eats and any symptoms or changes in mood or activity level that are not consistent with your child's behavior.

As you start to record the foods in the diary, you may not see immediate allergy symptoms, but, over time, causal relationships will begin to appear.

If you serve a food several days in a row, an allergy may show up. Foods or ingredients usually served daily, such as wheat, must be completely omitted when they are being tested on a trial avoidance diet.

Some symptoms to watch for include allergic shiners, a pallid appearance, and a tired feeling. These symptoms frequently can be traced to one or more food allergies. Once you have some suspect foods from information in the diary, you will probably have an idea what foods to avoid on the elimination diet.

Sometimes your diet diary results may show that several foods may be causing allergy. Therefore, the avoidance diet may not work until you eliminate all the suspect foods. If this is the case, a low allergy diet may be better to try. You can start out with low allergy foods and slowly add other foods back into the diet at three-week intervals.

Try an elimination diet when you have a pretty good idea as to the food your child is allergic to. Keep in mind the balance idea. You should try the diet when your child is not reacting to pollens, molds, or other allergies. If you find there is no good time, use a low allergy diet. A low allergy diet is also good when symptoms are a problem. There is supporting data that suggests that a low allergy diet may benefit any child having a flare-up of nonfood allergies. Sometimes an undetected food may aggravate an allergy flare-up.

For the elimination trial diet, take a suspect food out of the diet for three weeks. If there are no symptoms, add that food back in and try another one. If symptoms appear but are gone after a few days, continue to eliminate the food for the remainder of the three weeks. During the fourth week, serve that food several times. If symptoms reappear, take the food out of the diet for another three weeks. On the fourth week, reintroduce it and serve it several times. If the symptoms reappear a second time, you have found the allergy. Most parents find this process too tedious and prefer to use a low allergy diet instead.

On a low allergy diet, the child will eat low allergy foods for three weeks, or until symptom free. (Keep in mind that if other allergies are active, it may not be a good time to add suspect foods to the diet.) If the child has no symptoms, add one suspect food at a time at three-week intervals. If symptoms occur, take the last food added out of the diet for three weeks. Then reintroduce it. If the symptoms return, you have found a food allergy.

If you are bottle-feeding your baby, you and the doctor probably will start with a soy milk to avoid allergies. A child can, however, be allergic to soy but this is not too common.

If you are nursing your baby, your own diet is important. Some babies react to foods that the mother is eating. If the mother is on a low allergenic diet, there is less chance for trouble. If a nursing mother eats the same food every day, the baby may eventually get an allergy. Keep a good variety of foods in the diet to avoid this problem. However, it is very difficult to avoid wheat because it is in so many foods.

The following list identifies some low allergenic foods. Note that many of these foods are not in the usual diet and they may be low risk because they are uncommon. It would be wise to avoid eating any of them frequently.

- Cereals—barley, rice, soy
- Fruits—apricots, dates, grapefruit, lemons, peaches, pears, pineapple, prunes, rhubarb, tomatoes
- Meat—chicken, lamb, turkey
- Vegetables—artichoke, asparagus, beets, broccoli, carrots, chard, collards, kale, lettuce, lima beans, mustard greens, peas, spinach, squash, string beans, sweet potatoes, turnip greens, white potato, yam
- Other—baking powder, baking soda, creme of tartar, extract of lemon or orange, gelatin, maple syrup, olives (green), sesame oil, soy margarine, sugar (cane or beet), tapioca, white vinegar

47

vvvvvvvvvvvvvvvvvvvvvvvvvvvvvvvvvvvvvvvvvvvvvvvvvvvvvvvvvvvvvvvvvv

SLEEP PROBLEMS

Allergic children have the same sleep disorders as other children, except for certain problems associated with the allergic condition. These are sleep disturbances that occur because of discomfort or medication. If your child is deviating from expected childhood patterns, his allergies may be the cause.

It is not unusual for a normal child to have difficulty sleeping during the preschool years. Some children have trouble falling asleep; others walk or talk in their sleep. Many children fear that frightening figures—either human or animal—are in the room. Often, children are afraid to be alone. If your child experiences any of these behaviors, don't worry. Usually these problems are temporary. Bedtime rituals can help a child to settle down. These may include a bedtime story or song or two, a favorite stuffed toy, or just a reassuring snuggle and kiss.

Certain sleep behaviors can accompany certain ages. Most newborns sleep from eleven to eighteen hours a day. Sleeping for five- to six-hour stretches shows that your baby in maturing and will soon sleep through the night. Breast-fed babies take a little longer to reach this stage. Small babies may not reach the milestone of sleeping through the night as quickly as term or larger babies.

During the first to third years, some behavior problems are typically associated with sleep. Young children who have difficulty sleeping may just be crying for attention. They may wake several times a night crying or they may fight going to bed. Sometimes it is difficult to determine who is in control—the baby or the parent. These behaviors relate to developmental stages and may drive parents to seek professional help. It is important to maintain straightforward sleep patterns. Stick to the same bedtime and wake time. Use bedtime rituals such as a bath, tooth-brushing, or a story to help a child get in the mood.

Many children age three to five have sleep difficulties. Console yourself that this array of problems will pass. Some youngsters can't sleep; others won't sleep. Again, straightforward daily patterns are important.

When children reach grade school, most of them fall asleep quickly, sleep well, and are usually wide-awake and alert all day. They average from eight to ten hours of sleep at night. If your child is not sleeping well, review medications and sleep habits.

The teenager begins to sleep a little more, especially on weekends. It is not unusual for this age youngster to get sleepy during the day, or even to nap now and then. Biologically, the growth hormone is secreted during sleep. The teenagers' rapid growth during this period may require more sleep. This change in sleep patterns added to allergies may certainly increase the need for sleep. Recognize and accept this as normal. Teens may also start to vary their sleep times during these years. Encourage your child to stick to a regular schedule. If sleep disorders are a problem, consult your physician.

There are a few sleep problems that occur in allergic children. An earlier discussion in Key 44 (see page 122) covered how the mouth structures change because of mouth breathing. As the mouth structures narrow during development, the throat space at the back of the lower jaw also narrows. The angle of the shape of the lower jaw will influence the size of the opening in the throat. This space can become obstructed when the tongue and other soft tissues relax and fall back toward the throat.

When an allergic child has acquired these structure changes from mouth breathing, the result can be sleep apnea, a short absence of breathing during sleep. This temporary closure of the airway forces the blood oxygen level to drop during sleep. As a result, the individual with this condition feels sleepy during the day. If you notice that your child stops breathing for a few seconds and then gasps, this may be sleep apnea. Children with this problem often snore as air flutters the soft tissue aside. They are also usually sleepy during the day.

Enlarged tonsils and adenoids can obstruct breathing while the youngster sleeps. This is common in ages four to six. Around the age of seven, these tissues begin to shrink, and the problem subsides. Sometimes, enlargement will require the removal of the tonsils and adenoids.

If sleep apnea is a possibility, a workup in a sleep disorder center can pinpoint the cause and provide treatment recommendations. First, a device called an oximeter is placed on the child for one night to measure the amount of oxygen in the blood. Recordings are taken throughout the night to document the level of oxygen. There can be several causes if the level drops below normal. A sleep apnea workup consists of consultations with a dentist, an ear-nose-throat specialist, a pulmonologist, and a neurologist. These physicians will confer after each has studied the problem from his or her perspective. They will then recommend a treatment program.

The treatment options for obstructive sleep apnea depend upon what is blocking the airway. One method is to use continuous positive airway pressure (nasal CPAP). At bed-time a machine is attached to a mask worn by the patient. As room air is gently blown into the air passages, the pressure keeps the passages open. Another way sleep apnea is treated is by wearing a device called a jaw advancement device (JAD). The JAD moves the jaw forward, creating a larger airway. Sometimes loss of weight in an obese patient solves the prob-lem because soft tissue obstructing the airway disappears. With the young child, decongestants can keep the airway open just enough until the tonsils and adenoids shrink on their own. If the obstruction cannot be alleviated by these solution, surgery may be an option.

Colicky babies take longer to develop good sleep pat-terns. They are hard to comfort because they cry so much. Allergic babies with colic may not sleep through the night until they are six months of age or older.

Sometimes the first sign of asthma in a child is a dry cough while asleep. Frequently there are no other noticeable symptoms. Many children continue to sleep while coughing, but this symptom arouses them from deeper sleep. Since coughing limits restful sleep, these children are often tired or cranky during the day.

There are several reasons a child with asthma gets worse at night. Natural cortisol hormone levels are lowest during sleep in the early morning hours. These levels may be just low enough to provide an attack. Also, the lungs cannot work as well when a child lies down. Any child with breathing restriction will breathe better if sitting up.

Asthma attacks seldom occur during the early deep sleep stage called NREM (Non Rapid Eye Movement) sleep. Asth-matic children may not get to this deep sleep stage because the asthma keeps them in a higher sleep stage. In the later half the night, asthma occurs in both REM and NREM levels of sleep. This is probably related to low hormone levels. During REM sleep, the body is paralyzed, the brain is active, and the eyes move rapidly—hence the name, Rapid Eye Movement (REM). Dreams occur during the REM stage. Asthma may be triggered by dreams.

Some asthmatic children have difficulty getting good exchanges of air in and out of their lungs while they sleep. This form of sleep apnea may result from a combination of physical changes while asleep. Relaxed muscles, spasm of the airways, narrowed airways, and the fact that they cannot breathe as well while asleep are all factors.

Medication given to allergic children may stimulate them so they have difficulty sleeping. Steroids, decongestants, or theophylline can all stimulate behavior and keep children awake. Let your physician know about any sleeping difficulty. There are many combinations of medications. Sometimes you will have to try different medications before discovering the best one for your youngster. Each child's reactions are different.

Children with asthma require medication at bedtime to control attacks and ensure a good night's sleep. Lack of sleep will rob a child of daytime energy. Also, tired asthmatic children are more prone to daytime attacks. These children are most comfortable in a near-sitting position during sleep. Encourage your child to use a couple of pillows every night.

Children with allergic rhinitis may be unable to sleep because of nasal stuffiness. An antihistamine-decongestant with a side effect of drowsiness works well for them. Sometimes they also need to sleep on a couple of pillows.

As part of the natural steps toward independence, school-age children frequently start sleeping at a friend's home. As the parent of an allergic child, you need to be aware of the potential allergens and prepare the right medications. Give your child his or her pillow to take.

When your child sleeps away from home, it is not unusual for anxieties to appear. Support your child by telling her that her feelings are normal. Let her know that most people do not sleep well in a different bed and the usual comforts of home. A younger child might like to take along a favorite stuffed animal or toy.

Good sleep habits encourage a sound sleep and a refreshed feeling upon awakening. If your child is not sleeping well and you know the cause is not allergies or medications, review his sleeping habits.

Make certain your child gets enough sleep. Asthmatic children use a lot of energy when they have symptoms. They also tire easily. They will probably require a little more sleep if the quality of their sleep is poor.

Keep the daily patterns on roughly the same time schedule. Children then associate sleep with a certain hour and activity.

The foods your child eats and drinks play a role in sleeping habits. Some foods make you drowsy while others stimulate. Caffeine, for example, can stimulate for as long as seven hours. A big meal usually makes a person sleepy. Everyone has different effects from certain foods, whether or not an allergy is involved. If your child is food sensitive, you will gradually learn to know the foods that promote changes in behavior.

Exercise and play are essential to a good night's sleep. It has been found that physically active children, in many cases, will sleep the same amount as their peers, but the quality of the sleep may be better. Because exercise or play near bedtime may stimulate most children, try to encourage quiet activities in the evening.

Sending the child to his or her room for punishment may create negative feelings about sleep. Also, it is wise to avoid active play or stimulating games in the bedroom, particularly just before bedtime, if your child has a sleep problem. The bedroom should be only for sleeping.

The bedroom should be quiet. Even if your child is not awakened by noise, arousals from deeper sleep may occur, this resulting in a lower quality of sleep. Sometimes, white noise such as a fan or consistent street sounds can mask other noises. This may protect the quality of sleep. The console air cleaner used for many allergic children provides this comforting background noise.

The temperature of the room should be just right for your child. Whether it is warm or cool doesn't matter. If you have a child who coughs in cool air, keep the room warm enough to avoid symptoms. Room temperatures above 75 degrees result in a poorer quality of sleep.

The room should be well-ventilated. Ideally, there should be a minimum of four exchanges of room air each hour. You will not want to open a window, but be aware that a closed room may result in a high exposure to allergens or air pollutants, because of buildup. A console air cleaner will solve this problem.

Allergic children should sleep in a room with a humidity level of 25 to 50 percent. This provides a good environment for irritated respiratory passages.

The bed should be comfortable for your child. A slight sitting-up position and good, firm support for the body are important. Whether the mattress is innerspring or foam doesn't matter if a zippered dust free encasing covers it. There is increased humidity around most waterbeds. Because humidity encourages molds, these kinds of beds should be avoided. Launder all bedding a least once a month to control mites. Wash sheets and all pillow coverings more frequently, at least once a week.

Consistent patterns of care for any child will help develop good sleeping habits. It is important to conduct daily activities such as the bath or story-telling just before bed. Children need objects at night that are important to them throughout the day—a favorite toy or blanket, for example.

Keep sleep positive. Misperception is common with children, especially those between the ages of three and five. They may be having dreams that scare them and they may get the dreams mixed up with reality. Some may believe that if they do not sleep, they will not have bad dreams. Answer questions simply and encourage your child to talk to you about these kinds of worries.

If your child has excessive nightmares or repeated theme nightmares, talk to your pediatrician about them. A sleep center or psychologist referral may be necessary.

QUESTIONS AND ANSWERS

Q: I think two of our children have allergies. How can I find a good doctor? Do I need a specialist?
A: First talk to your doctor about your concerns. If he or she does not refer you to a specialist, contact any of the following for referrals. It is not unusual for a physician to miss allergy, because your child may not have symptoms at the office. Contact a branch of the American Lung Association or the Asthma and Allergy Foundation of America listed in the State Directory beginning on page 171). The National Jewish Center for Immunology and Respiratory Medicine, the National Allergy and Asthma Network, or the Asthma and Allergy Foundation of America all have 800 numbers listed under Organizations, Firms, and Associations (see page 163).

Q: My wife and I have allergies. We are expecting a child in six months. What can we do to prepare for a potentially allergic child?
A: You can condition your home by eliminating known common allergens. You have the time to condition the baby's bedroom so there are no sources for dust or dust mites. For example, enameled furniture is ideal for a small child. It resists dust and can take the spills and bumps of a small child. If possible, the floor should be wood coated with polyurethane. Use synthetic throw rugs and wash them once a month. The window should have an enameled shutter, a vertical blind or a vinyl shade. If you want to paper the walls, use vinyl-

coated or vinyl cloth covering. If you have forced air heating, consider closing off the ducts or vents to the bedroom. Small floor-level heating units can be installed under windows. They are not hot to touch, and they heat cold air from the window area.

Your wife should start to restrict her diet during the last months of pregnancy. Avoid daily eating of the same food and eat a low allergen diet. If she is going to nurse the baby, the diet restrictions should continue until the baby no longer nurses. If the baby is to be bottle-fed, the pediatrician will recommend a low allergenic formula. Most of them are soybean based.

Once your baby has started to eat, introduce low allergenic foods one at a time at intervals of two weeks or more. Start with rice, oat, and barley cereals.

Q: My son is allergic to milk. I worry that he will not get enough calcium.
A: Check with a nutritionist about the dietary needs for a child the age of your son. For most children, an antacid tablet like Tums each day will fulfill the requirement. Many vegetables are high in calcium.

Q: I change my baby frequently because she gets a terrible rash on her bottom. Could this be from a food allergy?
A: Food allergy may be one cause. Keep a diet diary for a few weeks to see if there is a relationship between the symptoms and some particular food. Watch for symptoms that appear one to two days after a food is eaten. If you are using cloth diapers, there may be soap residue in them. Sometimes the laundry softener causes irritation. Let your doctor know if the rash persists.

149

Q: Our daughter is five months old and has colic. I'm still nursing her and, in addition, I have her on rice and oat cereals, apples, and peaches.

A: Try to eat a low allergenic diet. It is worth a try. Also avoid eating the same food each day. In a case similar to yours, the mother drank apple juice each morning. When she stopped drinking it, the colic stopped. It may not be food. Some babies' gastrointestinal systems take up to a year to fully develop.

Q: My four-year-old son has had a mild skin inflammation since he was a baby. The back of his knees and the inside crease of his elbows are always red. He is constantly rubbing these areas.

A: Talk to your doctor about an allergy workup. It would be good to get these symptoms under control before he starts school. Once the allergens are identified, the physician can prescribe a skin care program.

Q: Our child's skin is weepy and red. Our family doctor tells us she will outgrow the condition. She is scratching every time I look at her.

A: Ask your doctor for a referral to an allergist or dermatologist. There is no way to tell if a child will outgrow eczema. An allergist may find other symptoms of allergy that you are unaware of.

Q: Often my neighbor will not let her son play with my son David. She says she doesn't want her boy to catch a cold. I have explained that David suffers from an allergy but she ignores me.

A: First, check your son's symptoms. Maybe it is his symptoms that offend her. Is he always coughing? Does he rub his nose because it is constantly running? You may not be aware of his mannerisms anymore. Sometimes we no longer see these behaviors. If his symptoms are under control, get some literature from an organization listed at the end of this book (see page 168) and share this material with her.

Q: Is it possible to know if your child is at risk for asthma?
A: Maybe. Lung functions can be done on an infant who is at risk by family history. Asthmatic babies may have lower-than-normal lung functions. Some of these children seem to have smaller airways. Mothers who smoked during pregnancy or who had poor nutrition also may have babies with smaller airways. This poses an additional risk factor for babies already at risk. History of the parents as well as any symptoms present early in life will give more of a clue.

Q: Now that inflammation, not spasm, is considered the most important aspect of chronic asthma, will the medications change?
A: They have already changed. Inhaled corticosteroids, powerful medicines to fight inflammation, are now the drug of choice. Once researchers learn about the chemicals causing inflammation, development of new medicines will follow.

Q: Are certain groups of children at higher risk for asthma than others?
A: Yes, children of low income families who live in the inner city have greater frequency of asthma.

Q: What causes asthma from exercise?
A: For years, researchers thought that exercise caused constriction of the airways. Recent evidence shows that airway swelling results from airway cooling and rewarming. Apparently, an excess flow of blood rushes toward airways cooled from exercise. Asthmatics have more blood vessels in the lung and have a greater flow of blood to the lungs during exercise.

Q: My husband teases our asthmatic son because he misses out on sports. I worry about our boy's self-esteem.

A: Insensitive teasing is not an unusual experience for an asthmatic child. Your son needs to talk about how he feels when Dad does this. If that doesn't work, see if your husband will attend a parents' support group meeting. Get information from organizations listed in the back of this book (see page 163). Also talk to your doctor about your child's restrictions. Some drugs taken prior to exercise can be helpful in controlling or preventing adverse reactions in asthmatic patients.

Q: Our daughter, age eight, uses a Peak Flow Meter to monitor her asthma, but we don't seem to make the right decisions quickly enough. She is having at least three attacks a month.

A: Excellent literature is available to help you. A copy of the highlights of the Expert Panel Report on the Management of Asthma, "Diagnosis and Management of Asthma," is available through the National Allergy and Asthma Network (see page 163). Most current books on asthma cover this problem.

Q: Our family doctor has treated all of our family for many years. It doesn't seem to concern him that our son has had pneumonia six times in the past three years. If I ask for a referral, I'm afraid I'll insult him.

A: A conscientious physician will not be insulted if you get a second opinion. If your own doctor will not refer you to an allergist, contact an organization listed in the back of this book (see page 163) for a referral. Underdiagnosis of asthma is prevalent. Pneumonia often is blamed when the problem is actually wheezing from asthma.

Q: We give our child theophylline as the doctor prescribes, but our daughter gets worse about two days after an attack begins. What are we doing wrong?

A: Inflammation is the major problem at this phase of the asthma attack. Theophylline is a bronchodilator that helps reduce inflammation. Your child needs a different medication routine once you notice warning signs. Talk to your doctor about getting a Peak Flow Meter to measure dropping lung functions.

Q: Our daughter requires oral corticosteroids often. We worry about long-term side effects.
A: Read the *Asthma Bulletin* of March 1991. It is an excellent report on the diagnosis and management of asthma. If your physician has not made changes in your child's medicine routine, discuss the fact. There are options. (You can request a reprint from Ted Klein & Co., 740 Broadway, New York, NY 20003.)

Q: My husband's work requires frequent moves. Each home we have moved to has had an allergy source problem for our child. How can we avoid some of these problems in the future?
A: Look for the major sources of allergy first. Where is the home located? From what direction does the prevailing wind blow? What is in the wind? You do not want to be near industry that contaminates the air. Once you have found the location, there are certain features that should be avoided or corrected when relocating a home.

- An old carpet and/or pad in a home will have to be replaced.
- The home history should show there has never been an indoor pet or a flood. Water damage from a water heater, an overflowing toilet, or a natural disaster results in mold problems.
- The home should be in good condition. If it is an old house, has it been well maintained? Newer homes are more desirable. Check for a plumbing leak under sinks.

- Can all wall surfaces be damp cleaned? Are they smooth so they will not hold dirt? Avoid homes with cork walls or natural wall coverings that are not sealed with vinyl or polyurethane.
- Is there a forced air heating system? Can a high-quality filter be installed?
- If the windows are covered with drapes, can they be removed? Can you substitute a treatment that is washable? For example, percale sheets can be used to make an attractive drapery. Smooth surface window coverings such as plastic vertical blinds, vinyl shades, or shutters are ideal.

Q: A local heating company installed an electronic air cleaner in our home. We have followed all the environment control recommendations. Twice a week, I find dust on the furniture.

A: Electronic air cleaners have some inherent problems. One is the installation itself. Transition ducts that go into and out of the cleaning-heating unit are necessary. Otherwise, the flow of air is not smooth, resulting in inefficient filtering. The speed of the blower is important for good operation. Sometimes the duct size or heating unit size is not right for the home. Unless the installer has experience with these units, you need an air conditioning engineer to figure what the requirement is for your home.

The fault might not lie with the electronic air cleaner. Do you leave windows open? Do you leave the filter blower on 24 hours a day? Do you wash the filter every month? Manufacturer's recommendations are not necessarily suitable for allergic people. There may also be a new allergen in the home.

Q: We live in an apartment building where cockroaches are a problem. My daughter has had allergy shots for two

years but still has significant problems. Are cockroaches common allergens?

A: There is a rising incidence of asthma in urban areas. The cockroach may be the cause. Rhinitis and skin rashes are also common symptoms. Presently, research is trying to identify specific cockroach proteins that cause the reaction. Skin tests are available. Long, cold winters keep human occupants at home and roaches inside; thus the exposure to roach allergen is higher. The warmer climates of the southern states also may encourage a heavier incidence of these pests.

Q: We have several areas in our home that mold is a problem. Does this mean our allergies will be worse?

A: Yes, the balance idea is operating. The more exposure you have, the better the chances are for reactions. If you live in a humid climate, purchase a dehumidifier if you do not have air conditioning. Keep the humidity level between 25 and 50 percent. Next, eliminate sources for molds. For example, if the tile grout in the bathroom is black, clean it thoroughly. Apply a mold inhibitor such as Zepheran and let it dry. Apply a mold silicon to the grout to create a resistant surface. Twice a month you must clean with Zepheran.

GLOSSARY

Adenoids glandlike tissue located in the back of the throat; They play a role in early life to stop pathogens from getting into the body.

Adrenaline see Epinephrine.

Adrenergic medication class of drugs that dilate the bronchioles to make air passages wider. They can be injected or inhaled.

Aerosol solution that is atomized into a fine mist for propelling medicines, household, and toiletry products into the air.

Air filter device to remove airborne contaminants.

Air purifier small device that filters a very small amount of air.

Allergen substance that triggers an allergic response; a substance foreign to the body.

Allergic dermatitis the medical term for eczema; inflammation of the skin caused by allergy.

Allergy hypersensitivity state acquired through exposure to a particular allergen.

Alveoli tiny, thin-walled air sac structures in the lung that allow the exchange of oxygen and carbon dioxide.

Anaphylaxis unusual or exaggerated reaction to a foreign substance in the body.

Antibody substance in the body that reacts with the entry of a foreign substance; it attaches to the foreign substance and causes a response.

Antigen substance that triggers the antigen-antibody response.

Asthma reversible condition of the lungs that causes recurrent attacks of shortness of breath, wheezing, coughing, and constriction due to spasm.

Atopy term that is interchangeable with hypersensitivity and allergy.

Autogenous self-generated; originated within the body; describes vaccine made from patient's own blood.

Beta-adrenergic class of drugs that dilate bronchioles to make air passages wider.

Beta 2 agonist class of drugs that act as bronchodilators.

Bromides chemical compound known to cause anaphylaxis in some people.

Bronchi the medical term for a branch of the windpipe; also called bronchial tubes; two airways that branch off the trachea, or windpipe.

Bronchial airway term for the lower respiratory tract where the windpipe branches into two airways, or bronchi.

Bronchiole small air passage in the lung.

Bronchitis inflammation of the air passages of the lungs.

Bronchodilator medication that relaxes the bronchial muscle and causes the bronchial airways to open.

Bronchospasm constriction of the air passages of the lung; a spasm in the bronchi.

Colic acute abdominal pain; a common ailment in newborns, thought to be result from an incompletely developed intestinal tract.

Conjunctivitis inflammation of the conjunctiva, a delicate membrane that lines the eyelids and covers the eyeball.

Corticosteroids hormones that have profound life-maintaining effects on the body; the term *steroids* is a short form of corticosteroids.

Cortisone hormone that helps regulate inflammation.

C-PAP device that blows room air through a mask worn by a sleeping person; air pressure keeps airways open.

Decongestant medication that has a drying effect on the upper respiratory passages.

Dermatitis inflammation of the skin.

Dyspnea difficult or labored breathing.

Eczema (allergic) inflammation of the skin with watery discharge and the development of scales and crusts; a result of scratching from itching.

Edema abnormally large amount of fluid in the intercellular tissue spaces of the body.

Electronic air cleaner filtering device that cleans air by blowing electronically charged airborne particles past a collector plate that has the opposite charge, resulting in a collection of the particles.

Environmentals term used to describe substances in the home, school, and work environment that cause allergies; plant and animal fibers that cause allergy.

Epinephrine term interchangeable with adrenaline; a powerful medication that increases blood pressure and stimulates the heart muscle to increase heart output; delivered by inhalation, topical application, or injection. In asthma, it causes bronchodilation.

Eustachian tube tube that equalizes air pressure between the throat and middle ear.

Expectorant medication thought to help in the expulsion of mucus from the lungs, bronchi, and trachea; a drug that liquifies secretions so they can be coughed up.

Extrinsic asthma asthma caused by substances outside the body, such as allergens.

Filters device used to filter airborne particles from the air; a simple mechanical filter, or charcoal filter. *See also* Electronic air cleaner; HEPA.

Flare term used to describe the red inflammation around a wheal during skin testing; the area of redness measured during skin testing.

Fungus term interchangeable with mold; a vegetable organism common in the environment.

Hay fever term used for allergic rhinitis, allergic hypersensitivity, and atopy.

HEPA High Efficiency Particulate Air filter; the most efficient filter for home use.

Histamine one of the chemicals released by mast cells when there is an antigen-antibody response; also released by ingesting certain foods such as strawberries in some allergic patients.

Hives skin eruption that may have many causes; characterized by bumpy eruptions. Allergy is a common cause.

Horse serum serum obtained from the blood of horses which have been injected with bacteria; known to cause anaphylaxis in some people.

Hymenoptera biological category of insects having four membranous wings, such as bees, wasps, ants, and other related forms.

Hypersensitivity abnormally sensitive reaction; a term interchangeable with allergy and atopy.

Hypotension low blood pressure.

IgE antibody associated with allergy.

Immunization the process of making a person immune to a disease.

Immunogenetics the branch of genetics concerned with the inheritance of antigenic or other characteristics related to the immune response.

Immunotherapy term interchangeable with allergy shots, and allergy injections.

Intrinsic asthma asthma caused by something inside the body—for example, asthma from sinus infections.

Lichenification the medical term for eczematous skin that

159

becomes scarred and thickened from constant scratching.

Mast cell tissue cell in the lining of the respiratory tract that releases chemicals after an antigen-antibody reaction.

Mold term interchangeable with fungus.

Mucus secretion produced by membranes that moistens and protects the body; mucus production from allergy can block passages or form plugs in the lungs.

Nebulizer device that sprays medicine so that it can be delivered deep into the lungs.

NREM Sleep non-REM sleep; relaxed or deep-sleep stage.

Off-gassing gases being given off into the air as part of the drying or aging process of new buildings or materials.

Oral steroid steroid given in pill or liquid form by mouth.

Peak flow meter hand device that measures how fast air is blown out of the lungs; helps to indicate when lung function is dropping or improving; also helpful for monitoring need for medications.

Pneumonia disease of the lungs that is characterized by inflammation and caused by viruses, bacteria, or chemicals.

Pollen microspores or the male element of plants and trees; part of the reproductive cycle.

Pollinosis allergic reaction in the body resulting from exposure to specific airborne pollens.

Polyp (nasal) growth arising from the lining of the nose into the nasal canal.

Rale abnormal respiratory sound heard through a stethoscope; often associated with pneumonia; sounds like a fine hair being plucked.

Rash temporary eruption on the skin, called urticaria.

REM the stage of sleep called Rapid Eye Movement. During this stage, the body is paralyzed, the eyes move rapidly, and dreaming occurs.

Rhinitis inflammation of the mucus membrane lining of the nose; also called *catarrhal, coryza, cold, hay fever.*

Rhonchi abnormal respiratory sound heard through a stethoscope; often associated with asthma; has a sound of congestion.

Serum the clear portion of blood when it is separated from its solid elements.

Shock term used for anaphylaxis; a condition of circulatory failure due to loss of circulating blood: the patient becomes pale and clammy, his blood pressure lowers, his pulse is rapid, and he sometimes loses consciousness.

Sleep apnea transient cessation of breathing, usually accompanied by a gasping sound; noisy breathing or snoring.

Sleep stages four levels of sleep, with REM and NREM alternating during the night. REM (short for rapid eye movement) typically begins about ninety minutes after sleep begins. There is intense brain activity and dreaming. Muscle activity is suppressed. REM represents about 20 to 25 percent of the total sleep of a young adult. The NREM (nonrapid eye movement) stage alternates with REM cycles. This phase lasts about ninety minutes, but REM sleep periods become progressively longer and NREM lighter as sleep continues through the night. Sleep stages include stage 1—the transition between wakefulness and sleep; stage 2—light sleep; stage 3—deeper sleep; and stage 4—deepest sleep. Sleepwalking or sleep terror attacks usually start in the later stages. Nightmares also occur more often during later stages of REM sleep.

Specificity term given to specific allergens causing an allergic reaction in one person; no two persons have the same allergies because each allergen is specific to a particular person.

Spirometer device that measures the amount of air inhaled and exhaled; used to measure the amount of airway obstruction in an asthmatic.

Steroid compound that has influence on the body's metabolism; more technically called *corticosteroid*; a drug that dilates bronchial tubes and decreases swelling; may protect against allergy; sometimes administered in combination with bronchodilator to enhance its effectiveness.

Theophylline drug that dilates or expands the bronchial tubes.

Tonsillectomy removal of the tonsil(s).

Tonsils small almond-shaped masses in the throat; composed of lymphoid tissue covered with mucus membranes. They protect the body from infection.

Trachea the windpipe; a pipelike structure in which air moves to and from the lungs.

Upper airways the nose, mouth, and throat. They warm and moisten air as it moves to the lungs.

Urticaria (allergic) the medical term for a rash or wheals that itch.

Wheal blisterlike skin eruption that occurs approximately ten minutes after an allergy skin test is applied to the skin; wheal and flare (red inflamed area), are measured during the skin testing.

Wheeze whistling sound made in breathing; sometimes heard without a stethoscope. The sound can be heard in the expiration of an asthmatic. The sound is produced when air pushes against swelling or congestion in the lungs.

ORGANIZATIONS, FIRMS, AND ASSOCIATIONS

T he following list includes profit and not-for-profit firms and organizations that provide assistance to the allergic person. Firms selling products for the home have been included to illustrate the type of products available to control allergies. There are many companies that sell these products. The product you pick should have the same specifications or better to control the environment.

Abbott Laboratories
Pharmaceutical Products Division
North Chicago, IL 60064
(800) 323-9100
    Booklets on allergy.

Allergy Control Products
96 Danbury Road
Ridgefield, CT 06877
(800) 422-DUST
    Products include allergen proof encasings, Allergy Control Solution (mite control).

Allergy Information Association
25 Poynter Drive, Suite 7
Weston, Ontario, Canada M9R 1K8
(414) 244-9312

A not-for-profit organization that offers allergy information to the general public and professionals; publishes a quarterly newsletter; reviews new books pertaining to allergy.

American Academy of Allergy and Immunology
611 East Wells Street
Milwaukee, WI 53202
(414) 272-6071
Physician and professional organization to advance the knowledge and practice of allergy and immunology; promotes knowledge of students and public; sponsors research.

American Allergy Association
P.O. Box 640
Menlo Park, CA 94026-7273
(415) 322-1663
Publishes handbook, provides information and health alerts, reviews books, offers recipes, answers questions.

American Lung Association
1740 Broadway
New York, NY 10019
(212) 315-8700
Offers booklets, asthma camps, support groups, classes.

Asthma and Allergy Foundation of America (AAFA)
1717 Massachusetts Avenue. N.W., Suite 305
Washington, DC 20036
(202) 265-0265   (800) 7-ASTHMA
Collects information for the public on new research; basic facts about asthma and allergies; produces and distributes pamphlets and bulletins; answers inquiries; supports research in allergy and the training of future allergists.

Asthma Care Association of America
611 E. Wells
Milwaukee, WI 53202
(800) 822-2762
　　Not-for-profit organization dedicated to supporting financially the care, treatment, and rehabilitation of persons with asthma and allergies; supports research and publishes the *Journal of Asthma*.

ATI (Air Techniques, Inc.)
11438 Cronridge Drive S. 2
Owings Mills, MD 2117
(410) 356-9941
　　Sells HEPA filter.

Bio-Tech Systems
P.O. Box 25380
Chicago, IL 60625
(800) 621-5545
　　Many products by catalog and educational literature.

Environmental Health Watch (EHW)
4115 Bridge Avenue
Cleveland, OH 44113
(216) 281-4663
　　Offers education on health effects of materials and chemicals in the environment.

Fisons Corporation
Marketing Division
Two Preston Court
Bedford, MA 01730
(617) 275-1000
　　Patient education literature (English and Spanish).

Health Services Consultants
2670 Del Mar Heights Road, #194
Del Mar, CA 92014
(619) 259-6146
FAX (619) 259-6169
   Consults, teaches, writes, and provides direct mail order of health education books and literature; includes allergy, allergy environment, and sleep disorders.

HiTech Filter Corporation of America
80 Myrtle Street
North Quincy, MA 02171
(800) 448-3249
   Sells filters.

Hollister-Stier
Miles Laboratory
400 Morgan Lane
West Haven, CT 06516
   Booklets on pollens, molds, allergy extracts, products.

Housing Resource Center (HRC)
1820 W. 48th Street
Cleveland, OH 44102
(216) 281-4663
   Provides consumers with home maintenance, repair, and improvement information; hot line and monthly newsletter.

Mothers of Asthmatics, Inc.,
See National Allergy and Asthma Network.

National Allergy and Asthma Network
3554 Chain Bridge Road, Suite 200
Fairfax, VA 22030-2709
(800) 878-4403

Maintains list of asthma support groups; provides information and literature; reviews books.

National Institute of Allergy and Infectious Diseases
NIH
Bethesda, MD 20205
Conducts research and research training for allergic and infectious diseases.

National Jewish Center for Immunology and Respiratory Medicine
1400 Jackson Street
Denver, CO 80206
(800) 423-8891
(800) 222-LUNG Nurse line
FAX 1-303-398-1125
Offers information, free brochures, physician and support group referrals, prevention treatment, rehabilitation, and research of immunological and respiratory diseases.

Nordyne, Inc.
1801 Park 270 Drive S. 600
St. Louis, MO 63146
(314) 878-6200
Sells Intertherm baseboard heaters.

Pharmacia Diagnostics
Division of Pharmacia, Inc.
800 Centennial Avenue
Piscataway, NJ 08854
Provides patient education literature on allergy.

Ross Laboratories
Division of Abbott Laboratories
Columbus, OH 43216
Provides patient education literature on allergy.

Searle Pharmaceuticals Inc.
Box 5110
Chicago, IL 60077
Provides patient education literature on allergy.

Tectronic Products Company, Inc.
6500 Badgley Road
East Syracuse, NY 13057
(315) 463-0240
(800) 227-1375
Sells electronic air cleaner, dehumidification equipment.

OTHER RESOURCES

Books and Literature on Allergies

Bock, S. Allan, M.D. *Food Allergy.* New York: Vantage Press, 1988. (Available through Asthma and Allergy Foundation of America).

Feldman, B. Robert, M.D. and David Carroll. *A Complete Book of Children's Allergies: A Guide for Parents,* New York: Random House, 1989. Available through Asthma and Allergy Foundation of America.

Plaut, Thomas F., M.D. *Children with Asthma, A Manual for Parents.* Amherst Mass.: Pedipress, 1989.

Literature For Children

American Lung Association. *See* State Directory.

National Allergy and Asthma Network. *See* Organizations, Firms, and Associations.

Books and Literature on Environment

"Air Purifiers" (reprint). *Consumer Reports,* February 1989.

American Lung Association. *See* State Directory.

Bachman, Judy L., *Allergy Environment Guidebook.* New York: Putnam, Perigee Books, 1990.

———. *Allergy Environment Control.* Booklet. *See* Health Services Consultants in Organizations, Firms, and Associations.

————. *Ensuring Clean Air*. Booklet. *See* Health Services Consultants in Organizations, Firms, and Associations.

National Allergy and Asthma Network. *See* Organizations, Firms, and Associations.

U.S. Environmental Protection Agency. *Indoor Air Facts #7, Residential Air Cleaners*. Reprint. Washington, D.C.: U.S. Government Printing Office, February 1990.

Books on Asthma

National Jewish Center for Immunology and Respiratory Medicine. *See* Organizations, Firms, and Associations.

Rudoff, Carol. *Asthma Resource Directory*. Available through National Allergy and Asthma Network. *See* Organizations, Firms, and Associations.

Sander, Nancy. *So You Have Asthma Too*. New York: Doubleday, 1989. Available through the National Allergy and Asthma Network. *See* Organizations, Firms, and Associations.

Spector, Sheldon, M.D. and Nancy Sander, eds. *Understanding Asthma: A Blueprint for Breathing*. Produced by the American College of Allergy and Immunology and available through the National Allergy and Asthma Network.

Weinstein, Allan M., M.D. *Asthma: The Complete Self-Management Guide to Asthma and Allergies for Patients and Their Families*. New York: Ballantine, Fawcett Crest Book, 1987. Available through National Allergy and Asthma Network.

General Information on Allergy

Rudoff, Carol. *Asthma Resource Directory*. Available through the National Allergy and Asthma Network.

STATE DIRECTORY

L istings for physician referral, research centers, support groups, and educational programs for all states are available through a number of organizations. Groups to contact include the National Jewish Center for Immunology and Respiratory Medicine and the National Allergy and Asthma Network (both listed in the section Organizations, Firms, and Associations), the American Lung Association (ALA), and the Asthma and Allergy Foundation of America (AAFA). Following is a directory of the ALA and AAFA, alphabetized by state.

Alabama
American Lung Association
  (ALA) of Alabama
900 S. 18th Street
Birmingham, AL 35209
(205) 933-8821

Alaska
ALA of Alaska
555 W. Northern Lights
  Boulevard, Suite 103
Anchorage, AK 99503-2501
(907) 276-5864

Arizona
Arizona Lung Association
102 W. McDowell Road
Phoenix, AZ 85003
(602) 258-7505

Arkansas
ALA of Arkansas
211 Batyrak Resources
  Drive
Little Rock, AR 72205
(501) 224-5864

California
Asthma and Allergy Foundation of America
AAFA Los Angeles Chapter
5225 Wilshire Boulevard,
  Suite 705
Los Angeles, CA 90036

ALA of California
424 Pendleton Way
Oakland, CA 94621-2189
(415) 638-5864

Colorado
ALA of Colorado
1600 Race Street
Denver, CO 80206-1198
(303) 388-4327

Connecticut
ALA of Connecticut
Eastern Branch
45 Ash Street
East Hartford, CT 06108
(203) 289-5401

Delaware
ALA of Delaware
1021 Gilpin Ave., Suite 202
Wilmington, DE 19806
(302) 655-7258

District of Columbia
ALA of the District of
    Columbia
475 H Street, N.W.
Washington, DC 20001
(202) 682-5864

Florida
ALA of Florida
5526 Arlington Road
Jacksonville, Florida
    32211-5216
(904) 743-2933

Asthma and Allergy Foun-
    dation of America
University Hospital
3100 E. Fletcher Avenue
Tampa, FL 33613-4688
(813) 972-7872

Georgia
ALA of Georgia
Perimeter and Northeast
    Branches
2452 Spring Road
Smyrna, GA 30080
(404) 434-8225

Hawaii
ALA of Hawaii
245 North Kukui Street
Honolulu, HI 96817
(808) 537-5966

Idaho
ALA of Idaho
1111 S. Orchard, Suite 245
Boise, ID 83705-1966
(208) 344-6567

Illinois
Asthma and Allergy Foun-
    dation of America
Greater Chicago Chapter
111 North Wabash, Suite 909
Chicago, IL 60602
(312) 346-0745

Chicago Lung Association
1440 W. Washington Boulevard
Chicago, IL 60607-1878
(312) 243-2000

Indiana
ALA of Indiana
9410 Priority Way, West Drive
Indianapolis, IN 46240-1470
(317) 573-3900

Iowa
ALA of Iowa
1025 Ashworth Road, Suite 410
West Des Moines, IA 50265
(515) 224-0800

Kansas
ALA of Kansas
4300 Drury Lane
Topeka, KS 66604-2419
(913) 272-9290

Kentucky
ALA of Kentucky
4100 Churchman Avenue
Louisville, KY 40215
(502) 363-2652

Louisiana
ALA of Louisiana
333 St. Charles Avenue,
   Suite 500
New Orleans, LA 70130-3180
(504) 523-5864

Maine
ALA of Maine
128 Sewall Street
Augusta, ME 04330
(207) 622-6394

Maryland
Asthma and Allergy Foun-
   dation of America
Maryland Chapter
5601 Loch Raven Boulevard
Baltimore, MD 21239-2995
(301) 532-4135

ALA of Maryland
1840 York Road,
Suites K–M
Timonium, MD 21093-5156
(301) 560-2120

Massachusetts
Asthma and Allergy Foun-
   dation of America
New England Chapter
220 Boylston Street,
   Suite 305A
Chestnut Hill, MA 02167
(617) 965-7771

ALA of Massachusetts
803 Summer Street,
Ground Floor
South Boston, MA
   02127-1609
(617) 269-9720

Michigan

ALA of Southeast Michigan
28860 West Ten Mile Road
Southfield, MI 48075
(313) 559-5100

Asthma and Allergy Foun-
dation of America
Michigan State Chapter
6900 Orchard Lake Road,
Suite 207
West Bloomfield, MI 48322
(313) 427-2202

Minnesota

ALA of Ramsey County
480 Concordia Avenue
St. Paul, MN 55103-2431
(612) 224-4901

Mississippi

Mississippi Lung Association
353 N. Mart Plaza
Jackson, MS 39206-9865
(601) 362-5453

Missouri

Asthma and Allergy Foun-
dation of America
Greater Kansas City Chapter
7905 E. 134th Terrace
Grandview, MO 64030
(816) 966-8164

ALA of Eastern Missouri
1118 Hampton Avenue

St. Louis, MO 63139-3196
(314) 645-5505

Asthma and Allergy Foun-
dation of America
St. Louis Area Chapter
222 S. Central, Suite 600
St. Louis, MO 63105
(314) 726-6866

Montana

ALA of Montana
Christmas Seal Building
825 Helena Avenue
Helena, MT 59601
(406) 442-6556

Nebraska

ALA of Nebraska
401 E. Gold Coast Road,
Suite 331
Omaha, NE 68128-4746
(402) 331-9000

Asthma and Allergy Foun-
dation of America
Missouri Valley Chapter
3612 S. 105th Street
Omaha, NE 68124
(402) 393-4664

Nevada

ALA of Nevada
6119 Ridgeview Court
Reno, NV 85905
(702) 829-5864

174

New Hampshire
ALA of New Hampshire
456 Beech Street
Manchester, NH 03103
(603) 669-2411

New Jersey
ALA of New Jersey
1600 Route 22 East
Union, NJ 07083
(908) 9340

New Mexico
ALA of New Mexico
216 Truman N.E.
Albuquerque, NM 87108
(505) 265-0732

New York
ALA of New York State
8 Mountain View Avenue
Albany, NY 12205-2899
(518) 459-4197

North Carolina
ALA of North Carolina
Research Triangle Region
800 St. Mary's Street
Raleigh, NC 27605-0394
(919) 834-8235

North Dakota
ALA of North Dakota
212 N. 2nd Street
Bismarck, ND 58501
(701) 223-5613

Ohio
ALA of Ohio
1700 Arlingate Lane
Columbus, OH 43228
(614) 279-1700

Oklahoma
ALA of Oklahoma
2442 N. Walnut
Oklahoma City, OK 73105
(405) 524-8471

Oregon
ALA of Oregon
1776 S.W. Madison
Portland, OR 97205
(503) 224-5145

Pennsylvania
ALA of Pennsylvania
4807 Jonestown Road, Suite 251
Harrisburg, PA 17109
(717) 540-8506

Asthma and Allergy Foun-
    dation of America
Southeast Pennsylvania Chapter
P.O. Box 249
Plymouth Meeting, PA 19462
(215) 825-0582

Rhode Island
Rhode Island Lung Asso-
    ciation
10 Abbott Park Place
Providence, RI 02903-3703
(401) 421-6487

South Carolina
ALA of South Carolina
Midlands Branch
1817 Gadsden Street
Columbia, SC 29201
(803) 779-0540

South Dakota
South Dakota Lung Association
208 E 13th Street
Sioux Falls, SD 57102-1099
(605) 336-7222

Tennessee
ALA of Tennessee
Middle Tennessee Region
1808 West End Avenue,
   Suite 514
Nashville TN 37203
(615) 329-2674

Texas
ALA of Texas
3520 Executive Center
   Drive, Suite G100
Austin, TX 78731-1698
(512) 343-0502

Utah
ALA of Utah
1930 South 1100 East
Salt Lake City, UT
   84106-2317
(801) 484-4456

Vermont
Vermont Lung Association
30 Farrell Street
South Burlington, VT 05403
(802) 863-6817

Virginia
ALA of Virginia
311 South Boulevard
Richmond, VA 23220
(804) 355-3295

Washington
ALA of Washington
2625 3rd Avenue
Seattle, WA 98121-1213
(206) 441-5100

West Virginia
ALA of West Virginia
415 Dickinson Street
Charleston, WV 25301
(304) 342-6600

Wisconsin
ALA of Wisconsin
1330 N.113 Street, Suite 190
Milwaukee, WI 53226-3212
(414) 258-9100

Wyoming
ALA of Wyoming
415 E. Pershing Boulevard
Cheyenne, WY 82001
(307) 638-6342

INDEX